THE
EVERYTHING®
GUIDE TO MANAGING AND REVERSING PRE-DIABETES,
2ND EDITION

Dear Reader,

The news that you have pre-diabetes is something you should take seriously. Whether you have just heard this news, or you have known for a while, you probably realize that healthy eating and lifestyle changes are necessary parts of your future. *The Everything® Guide to Managing and Reversing Pre-Diabetes, 2nd Edition* is a resource designed to help you make the transition to a healthier lifestyle and way of eating.

As a dietitian and diabetes educator in private practice, I've had many new clients come to my office who have just learned they have pre-diabetes. Invariably there is much confusion over the question "What can I eat?" There is often anticipation of hearing that favorite foods are going to be taken away. After we discuss what pre-diabetes is and how to make healthy eating and lifestyle choices, most of my clients leave their first appointments feeling pleasantly surprised. They have learned that managing pre-diabetes is about common sense and moderation, not deprivation.

It is my sincere hope that the information in this book helps you on your path to managing your pre-diabetes. Your perseverance and follow-through with the recommendations may make it possible to reverse the pre-diabetes. Taking action is the first step toward halting the progression of pre-diabetes.

For me, developing and testing the recipes found in this book has been a very enjoyable extension of my work as a Certified Diabetes Educator. When recipes result in great-tasting foods, cooking becomes a pleasure. I hope you will come away feeling pleasantly surprised!

Gretchen Scalpi, RD, CDN, CDE

Welcome to the EVERYTHING® Series!

These handy, accessible books give you all you need to tackle a difficult project, gain a new hobby, comprehend a fascinating topic, prepare for an exam, or even brush up on something you learned back in school but have since forgotten.

You can choose to read an Everything® book from cover to cover or just pick out the information you want from our four useful boxes: e-questions, e-facts, e-alerts, and e-ssentials.

We give you everything you need to know on the subject, but throw in a lot of fun stuff along the way, too.

We now have more than 400 Everything® books in print, spanning such wide-ranging categories as weddings, pregnancy, cooking, music instruction, foreign language, crafts, pets, New Age, and so much more. When you're done reading them all, you can finally say you know Everything®!

QUESTION

Answers to common questions

FACT

Important snippets of information

ALERT

Urgent warnings

ESSENTIAL

Quick handy tips

PUBLISHER Karen Cooper

MANAGING EDITOR, EVERYTHING® SERIES Lisa Laing

COPY CHIEF Casey Ebert

ASSOCIATE PRODUCTION EDITOR Mary Beth Dolan

ACQUISITIONS EDITOR Lisa Laing

DEVELOPMENT EDITOR Brett Palana-Shanahan

EVERYTHING® SERIES COVER DESIGNER Erin Alexander

Visit the entire Everything® series at www.everything.com

THE EVERYTHING® GUIDE TO MANAGING AND REVERSING PRE-DIABETES

2ND EDITION

Your complete guide to treating
pre-diabetes symptoms

Gretchen Scalpi, RD, CDN, CDE
Foreword by Robert Vigersky, MD

Adams Media
New York London Toronto Sydney New Delhi

*To my all of my clients with pre-diabetes and
diabetes who have taught me so much about the
challenges and rewards of managing their health.*

Adams Media
An Imprint of Simon & Schuster, Inc.
100 Technology Center Drive
Stoughton, MA 02072

An Everything® Series Book.
Everything® and everything.com® are registered trademarks of Simon & Schuster, Inc.

ADAMS MEDIA and colophon are trademarks of Simon and Schuster.

For information about special discounts for bulk purchases, please contact Simon &
Schuster Special Sales at 1-866-506-1949 or business@simonandschuster.com.

The Simon & Schuster Speakers Bureau can bring authors to your live event. For more
information or to book an event contact the Simon & Schuster Speakers Bureau at 1-866-
248-3049 or visit our website at www.simonspeakers.com.

Manufactured in the United States of America

14 2023

Library of Congress Cataloging-in-Publication Data has been applied for.

ISBN 978-1-4405-5761-3
ISBN 978-1-4405-5762-0 (ebook)

Contents

Acknowledgments

I would like to thank the staff at Adams Media for their advice and technical support.

A special thank you to my husband John, who for thirty-nine years has supported all of my career endeavors by making my life easier during busy times. He has always been willing to sample the many new recipes that made their way to the dinner table.

In remembrance and appreciation of my dear friend Jon Hines, who shared his wonderfully creative ideas, great food, and everlasting friendship.

Foreword

WE ARE IN THE midst of a world-wide tsunami of obesity and diabetes—or "diabesity" as it is commonly referred to because the two conditions are closely linked. Both obesity and diabetes have early stages, called "over-weight" and "pre-diabetes," that can be successfully targeted to prevent their progression to these more serious diagnoses.

The urgency of the problem is emphasized by an ugly statistic: nearly 79 million Americans have pre-diabetes as of 2010, yet only 10 percent have been told they have it. Knowing your diagnosis and doing something about it is critical. First and foremost, ask you healthcare provider to check you for pre-diabetes and diabetes particularly if you are in one of the high risk groups as outlined in the first chapter of this book. Don't wait for symptoms to appear since they often come late in the disease.

As a practicing endocrinologist, I regularly see patients ravaged by these dreaded diabetic complications—blindness, amputations, kidney failure, and heart disease—who learned they had pre-diabetes or diabetes too late. Even if patients are successful in preventing this damage, it is likely to have caused substantial changes in their lives and lifestyles (and those of their loved ones). One reason for this is that patients with diabetes take an average of eight medications a day (one of which is often insulin) to control their blood sugar and its commonly associated conditions of high blood pressure and high cholesterol. Much of this could have been avoided if they had asked their healthcare provider to check for pre-diabetes and then followed the advice about how to manage it.

Gretchen Scalpi has written a easily readable yet compelling and lucid account of the causes and management of pre-diabetes that makes it both enjoyable and rewarding to engage in the "ounces of prevention" that it takes to stay healthy.

A book that helps you tackle this important personal health (and public health) issue couldn't be timelier since it is predicted that one of every three

Americans born today will develop diabetes as an adult unless we find a way to stem this epidemic. This second edition also addresses the important issues of childhood/teenage obesity and pre-diabetes, which are rising at a startling rate, and includes age-appropriate strategies to deal with these problems.

There are also important new and expanded sections with advice on issues specific to women including gestation diabetes and polycystic ovary syndrome, both of which are directly related to obesity and pre-diabetes. Moreover, the recommendations in this book are applicable even to those who don't yet have pre-diabetes—call it "pre-pre-diabetes." These are people who have blood sugars that, although in the "normal" range, are really not normal. This is because the blood sugar cutoffs to distinguish diabetes from pre-diabetes (126mg/dl versus 125mg/dl) and pre-diabetes from normal (100mg/dl versus 99mg/dl) are arbitrary. In fact, we know that the risk of diabetes and cardiovascular disease increases continuously beginning with blood sugars as low as 80mg/dl—a level that may exist for years before the diagnosis of pre-diabetes. This explains why even some patients who are newly diagnosed with diabetes already have some diabetic complications—they have had years of exposure to sugars that are physiologically abnormal despite what the laboratory's "normal" range is showing.

Strategies focused on changing one's lifestyle are essential to the prevention and/or delay of diabetes particularly since there are no medications that are approved for this purpose. Such strategies, which have been proven in large clinical trials to be effective in delaying the onset of diabetes, are laid out in a very practical and easily understandable format in this book. It is quite appropriate that Chapter 4 on exercise precedes a chapter on diet management since there is accumulating evidence that exercise not only burns off calories while you are doing it but also stimulates your cells to turn on their metabolism and burn sugar for hours afterward giving you "more bang for the buck." There are many useful tips on how to get started with an exercise program, but one that should hit home to many is the advice to avoid buying a piece of exercise equipment at the outset. I have always fantasized that in retirement I'll open a used exercise equipment store stocked with my patients' bicycles, weight machines, etc., that were used enthusiastically for a few weeks but ultimately ended up as expensive clothes hangers or just dust collectors. Start simply and cheaply. Make a commitment in your time before you unnecessarily spend your hard-earned money.

Chapter 5 is no less important in providing a sensible approach to choosing the right foods whether eating at home or in a restaurant. The bonus is that there are delicious recipes that apply the principles of these healthy choices. As a diabetes educator, Ms. Scalpi clearly believes that knowledge is power. Read this book and take advantage of your acquired power to stay healthy!

ROBERT A. VIGERSKY, MD
Director, Diabetes Institute of the Walter Reed
National Military Medical Center
Past President of The Endocrine Society

Introduction

IF YOU ARE READING this book, odds are that you have concerns about the fact that you or a loved one has pre-diabetes. Pre-diabetes often has no symptoms; therefore, one may not realize he has the condition. Many people know that they need to "do something" about their weight or lack of exercise, but until something goes wrong there seems no need for urgency. Once you have learned that you or a loved one has pre-diabetes, however, there is an urgency to take action.

Managing pre-diabetes means understanding what it is and what to do about it. The more you understand, the better you can take action to reverse it or minimize your risk of developing type 2 diabetes. Luckily, by reading this book and putting some ideas into practice, you will have taken the first steps toward learning all you can about managing and reversing pre-diabetes.

Before delving into the specifics of pre-diabetes, here's a quick overview of diabetes. Once you understand more about diabetes, you will see the connection to pre-diabetes and why action on your part should not be put off.

Diabetes Mellitus

Every time you eat, your body converts the foods you consume into glucose (sugar). Insulin is a hormone the body makes that enables the glucose to get into cells, and the glucose is used for energy. People with diabetes either lack sufficient amounts of insulin or are unable to use the insulin they make. When insulin is absent or ineffective, the body is unable to get energy into cells and the level of glucose in the blood increases. To put it simply, your blood sugar level is too high. Genetics, obesity, and lack of exercise appear to be causal factors in most cases of diabetes. There are also several different types of diabetes.

Type 1 Diabetes

Approximately 5–10 percent of known cases of diabetes are classified as type 1 diabetes. Type 1 diabetes was formerly referred to as juvenile-onset diabetes because the onset typically occurs before the age of thirty. Type 1 diabetes is an autoimmune disorder that is thought to develop when stress factors (such as a viral infection) damage or destroy the beta cells of the pancreas. The person with type 1 diabetes is always dependent upon insulin because his or her pancreas no longer produces insulin. Type 1 diabetes is usually not associated with obesity or lack of exercise. Our discussion of pre-diabetes in this book will be focused on type 2 diabetes rather than type 1 diabetes.

Type 2 Diabetes

The vast majority of individuals who have diabetes have type 2 diabetes. For most people with type 2 diabetes, the pancreas still produces insulin, but it is being produced in insufficient amounts, or the body simply is unable to use the insulin in an efficient way.

Most people with type 2 diabetes are diagnosed in mid to late adulthood. Unfortunately, with the growing prevalence of obesity among children, we are now seeing children and young adults with type 2 diabetes as well.

Type 2 diabetes is often related to a sedentary lifestyle and an overweight or obese status. It is important to understand that diabetes is a disease that will progress, and while it can be controlled, it cannot be cured. Over time many people with type 2 diabetes may require oral medications and/or insulin to effectively treat and manage the disease. If untreated, a person with pre-diabetes may go on to develop type 2 diabetes.

Gestational Diabetes

Gestational diabetes is similar to type 2 diabetes because the body still makes insulin; however, a hormone secreted by the placenta interferes with the action of insulin. The result is elevated blood glucose levels usually starting around the twenty-fourth to twenty-eighth week of the pregnancy. In most cases, a pregnant woman's blood glucose returns to normal after the delivery of the baby and the diabetes is gone. A woman who has had gestational diabetes in the past has an increased risk of developing type 2 diabetes at a later time in her life, especially if she remains overweight or sedentary.

Seven Self-Care Behaviors

Managing diabetes and pre-diabetes is all about making lifestyle changes. The American Association of Diabetes Educators believes that utilizing principles of the Seven Self-Care Behaviors is an effective way to make positive changes in lifestyle. The self-care behaviors listed below apply to those with pre-diabetes and diabetes:

THE SEVEN SELF-CARE BEHAVIORS

1. **Healthy Eating:** Make healthy food choices, understand portion sizes, and learn the best times to eat.
2. **Being Active:** Include regular activity for overall fitness, weight management, and blood glucose control.
3. **Monitoring:** Daily self-monitoring of blood glucose to assess how food, physical activity, and medications are working.
4. **Taking Medication:** Understand how medications work and when to take them.
5. **Problem Solving:** Know how to problem-solve. For example, a high or low blood glucose episode could require the ability to make a quick decision about food, activity, or medication.
6. **Reducing Risks:** Effective risk reduction behaviors such as smoking cessation and regular eye exams are examples of self-care that reduce risk of complications.
7. **Healthy Coping:** Good coping skills that deal with the challenges of diabetes help people stay motivated to keep their diabetes in control.

As you read this book, you will find practical tools to empower you to take control of your health. Taking control means having an effective action plan that you can live with and is achievable. With practical tools and an effective plan, you have been given an opportunity to prevent or delay the onset of type 2 diabetes. Take it!

CHAPTER 1

What Is Pre-Diabetes?

Your doctor has just told you that you or your loved one has pre-diabetes. Your initial reaction might have been shock, anger, or a feeling of helplessness. Perhaps you knew something was not quite right all along, but you had put off going to the doctor and tried to put the whole thing out of your mind. Whatever the case, you are now faced with a medical diagnosis that has the potential to be serious. Many people in this situation find that they have not been given any tangible instructions about what pre-diabetes means or what to do about it. The best place to start is to learn more about pre-diabetes, then put together your action plan to stop pre-diabetes in its tracks.

The Pre-Diabetes Epidemic in America

The most recent data from the National Diabetes Fact Sheet 2011 states there are an estimated 79 million American adults aged twenty years or older with pre-diabetes. Yes, you read that correctly: 79 million Americans! The estimated numbers are growing annually, in large part because the presence of pre-diabetes is linked to America's other serious health problem: overweight and obesity. Being overweight and having elevated blood sugar (either diabetes or pre-diabetes) tend to go hand in hand. Blood sugar that fluctuates too high or too low throughout the day has a direct influence on your hunger level, snacking habits, and overeating. If your blood sugar is too low, you may eat too much food. If you eat too much food, over time you gain weight. When you gain too much weight, you are setting the stage for developing pre-diabetes, or worse yet, diabetes.

If you are obese, your risk for developing diabetes is far greater than for someone whose weight is normal. Today roughly two out of every three American adults are heavy enough to be considered overweight or obese. Data from the National Health and Nutrition Examination Survey 2009–2010 (Centers for Disease Control and Prevention) indicates that 35.7 percent of adults in the United States were obese. One thing is very clear about this trend: It means that the number of people who will develop diabetes or pre-diabetes is going to continue to grow.

QUESTION

How does the CDC determine statistics for pre-diabetes?
According to the National Diabetes Fact Sheet 2011, diabetes affects 25.8 million people. Based on fasting glucose or hemoglobin A1c levels, in 2005–2008, 35 percent of adults twenty years or older were found to have pre-diabetes. Applying this percentage to the 2010 census yields the estimated 79 million American adults with pre-diabetes.

Our Younger Generations: What's Going On?

The media is filled with reports about the troubling increase of childhood and adolescent obesity. Overweight and obesity among children has been steadily increasing over the past four decades. In 1971, 4 percent of children ages six to eleven were obese; in 2005, that percentage had increased to 17.4 percent! In the age group of twelve to nineteen, the obesity rate increase was similar: 6.1 percent in 1971 to 17.9 percent in 2005. Today, there are many more overweight school-age children, whereas several decades ago, overweight or obese children were much less common.

What are the key reasons for this alarming increase? There are several factors. Our food habits have changed a lot over the past several decades. Most of today's children have exposure to a vast array of fast foods, convenience foods, and empty-calorie snack foods. Tempting foods are readily available everywhere and at any time. Children learn about fast foods, soft drinks, and snacks through repeated exposure to television and other forms of advertising. Grocery store aisles are filled with sweetened foods, cereals, beverages, candies, and even kid-specific versions of yogurt with cookie and candy toppings. Food products are targeted and marketed specifically to children. A quick review of Saturday morning cartoons can teach you something about how products are pitched to children. It comes as no surprise that children want and request foods or snacks that have been heavily marketed to them.

In addition, today's families rely much more on eating out. Fast foods, convenience, or take-out foods are consumed often. The reasons for eating out more often include lack of time or energy to plan healthy meals at home, or not understanding the importance of good nutrition. Parents want to do the right thing for their children, but fast-paced lifestyles have gotten in the way. For some, family dinner at home has been replaced by dinner in the car at the drive-through. Unfortunately, many children learn to make strong associations with foods and beverages that have little nutritional value, and in fact contribute to obesity. Like adults, overweight or obese children are far more likely to develop pre-diabetes or type 2 diabetes.

What Makes Pre-Diabetes Different from Type 2 Diabetes?

The term *pre-diabetes* was introduced by the American Diabetes Association in 2002 as a way to more clearly convey a state that is between normal blood sugar and type 2 diabetes. In the past your doctor may have diagnosed you with "borderline diabetes." Other statements that have been used (euphemistically) are "your blood sugar is a little high" or "you have a touch of sugar." These words provide little meaning to the person hearing them, and they certainly do not express the urgent need to do something about the situation. Pre-diabetes *is* defined by tangible parameters, namely the results of blood glucose tests:

- Normal is defined as: fasting blood glucose (Fasting blood glucose means level of sugar in the blood after a ten- to twelve-hour fast and reflects what blood sugar is at the moment it is drawn) is less than 100mg/dl (milligrams per deciliter) and a glucose level less than 140mg/dl two hours after eating.
- Pre-diabetes is defined as: fasting blood glucose between 100–125mg/dl and a glucose level between 140–190mg/dl two hours after eating.
- Diabetes is defined as: fasting blood glucose of 126mg/dl or higher or a blood glucose greater than 200mg/dl two hours after eating.

ESSENTIAL

To confirm a diagnosis of either pre-diabetes or diabetes, the blood glucose levels must be elevated and within defined lab results at least two times. If your lab results indicated high glucose readings during an initial test, your doctor should repeat the test a second time to see whether the results are the same.

When you have pre-diabetes, your blood sugar level is higher than normal, but it's not yet high enough to be classified as type 2 diabetes. Pre-diabetes means that you are on your way to developing diabetes if there are no interventions on your part. One very important fact to understand is that progressing to type 2 diabetes is not inevitable. There is a great deal that you can do to reverse pre-diabetes and bring your blood sugar level back to a normal range. A diagnosis of type 2 diabetes, on the other hand, is permanent. While there is much that can be done to control diabetes, it is important to realize that type 2 diabetes does not go away. In spite of everything you have read so far, if you have received a diagnosis of pre-diabetes, there is some good news. You have received a wake-up call and been given an opportunity to improve your health, lose weight, and make healthy lifestyle changes. If you take action, you can prevent, or at the very least halt, the progression to a serious, permanent disease.

Risk Factors and Symptoms

In addition to laboratory results for fasting and post-meal glucose levels, there are other risk factors to consider. The factors that increase your risk of type 2 diabetes are the same risk factors for pre-diabetes. Check to see whether you fit any of these:

- **Age:** Forty-five years old or older
- **Family history:** A parent or sibling with type 2 diabetes
- **Weight:** Overweight or obese (the primary risk factor for pre-diabetes)
- **Race/ethnic background:** Hispanic, American Indian, African American, Asian American, and Pacific Islander
- **Exercise:** Inactive and sedentary lifestyle
- **Pregnancy:** Gestational diabetes during a past pregnancy
- **Other conditions:** Polycystic ovary syndrome (PCOS)
- **Other conditions:** Inadequate sleep of fewer than 5.5 hours nightly

Risk factors are used to determine increased susceptibility. The more risk factors present in your profile, the greater the risk for developing pre-diabetes or diabetes.

What about Symptoms?

Symptoms associated with pre-diabetes can be nonexistent or indistinguishable from other causes. Early symptoms of pre-diabetes are so common, in fact, that many people barely notice them at all, or think that what they are feeling is "normal." The symptoms are vague, very common, and rarely interfere with daily activities. However, sometimes the red flags associated with type 2 diabetes begin to appear, such as:

- Increased thirst
- Frequent urination
- Fatigue that doesn't improve with more sleep
- Blurred vision that may come and go

It is often not until several symptoms are noticed that a person begins to realize that things are not quite right.

What is acanthosis nigricans?
Acanthosis nigricans is one of the few early signs of pre-diabetes and may be noticed by an individual. It is characterized by a darkening of skin that typically affects the neck, armpits, elbows, knees, or knuckles. The darkening of pigment around these areas of the body can be an early sign of glucose abnormality. The condition does not affect everyone, and is found most often in native Americans, African Americans, and Hispanics. While there is no specific treatment for acanthosis nigricans, treatment of underlying conditions, such as a glucose abnormality, may restore some of the normal color to affected areas of skin.

Why You Can't Ignore Pre-Diabetes

Not that long ago, doctors did not routinely screen for, or treat, pre-diabetes aggressively. People who had glucose readings that were higher than normal but were not yet diabetic seldom received advice to reduce their risk of developing type 2 diabetes. That was before there was a good understanding about how glucose levels in the pre-diabetic range could actually cause vascular damage or other complications. Today we know that waiting until someone has progressed to diabetes could mean that complications have already begun to take hold. For this reason, the fasting blood glucose cutoff for pre-diabetes was lowered from 140mg/dl to 125mg/dl. Today a *normal* fasting blood glucose is below 100mg/dl. The lowering of the blood glucose ranges have helped detect poor glucose tolerance in many people, much earlier.

If you've been informed that you have pre-diabetes, you can be grateful that you know about the problem now, at an early stage. The most compelling reason to address pre-diabetes is your ability to halt or slow the progression to diabetes. If the right things are done at an early stage, a person may be able to reverse the pre-diabetic state. Even if you are only able to slow down the eventual progression to diabetes, you can minimize your risk for developing diabetic complications, such as heart disease, kidney failure, or diabetic retinopathy.

ALERT

People who do nothing and allow their blood sugar to creep up over time may already be developing some of the complications associated with diabetes. According to the American Diabetes Association, some long-term damage to the body, especially the heart and circulatory system, may already be occurring during pre-diabetes. Taking actions early on can help you prevent diabetic complications.

It is important to understand that diabetes does not occur suddenly. For most people, the progression from normal to pre-diabetic then to diabetic can take a number of years. The longer your body experiences high glucose levels, the greater your chance of developing diabetes-related complications.

CHAPTER 2

Diagnosing Pre-Diabetes

If you are trying to determine whether you have pre-diabetes, or monitor your condition after you have been diagnosed, you will need to have some information about your health. This information includes lab tests, blood pressure, and other measurements such as height, weight, and waist circumference. Your prior health history provides additional clues in the determination of pre-diabetes or diabetes.

Getting Tested and Understanding the Results

A fasting blood glucose test is the first essential test that provides a clue about the possibility of pre-diabetes. This is a simple blood test where a sample of blood is drawn first thing in the morning after an overnight fast. A fasting blood glucose between 100 and 125mg/dl on more than one occasion is an indicator for pre-diabetes. Some doctors prefer using a glucose challenge rather than a fasting test. In this case, you are given a glucose drink that provides 75 grams of glucose. Blood is drawn two hours after taking the drink and then the blood glucose is measured.

With this test, a blood glucose result of 140–199mg/dl two hours after taking 75 grams of glucose (on more than one occasion) indicates pre-diabetes. Two-hour readings that are above 200mg/dl on more than one occasion indicate diabetes.

ESSENTIAL

A fasting blood glucose test means just that: fasting. If you are having your blood test in the morning, you should not have anything to eat or drink (besides water) after midnight. Refrain from doing exercise before your test, because that could affect your reading, providing an inaccurate result.

What Other Blood Tests Are Important?

There are several other useful tests that can be helpful, not only for determining pre-diabetes, but also for monitoring it once diagnosed.

When a fasting glucose test or two-hour glucose challenge is done, the reading provides a result for that moment in time. Because your glucose can vary a great deal throughout the day, these tests do not provide information about what your blood sugar is at other times of the day. That is why a test called the hemoglobin A1c is done, particularly when pre-diabetes or diabetes is suspected. Hemoglobin is a substance found in red blood cells that carries oxygen from the lungs to all cells in the body. When hemoglobin binds with glucose, an irreversible compound, glycated hemoglobin (or glycohemoglobin), is formed. The A1c portion of glycated hemoglobin is the easiest and largest portion of this compound to measure. A person with higher blood glucose has more glycated hemoglobin formed than someone with normal blood glucose. Hemoglobin found in red blood cells lasts for sixty to ninety days. As a result, when hemoglobin A1c is measured, a fairly accurate reflection of your average blood glucose levels over the last sixty to ninety days can be determined. A hemoglobin A1c between 6 and 7 percent matches average glucose levels typically found in pre-diabetes. Monitoring your hemoglobin A1c and keeping it below 6 percent should be part of your action plan. Your doctor will monitor your hemoglobin A1c every three to six months by ordering a blood test.

QUESTION

Do I need a glucose meter even if I don't have diabetes?
If you have been diagnosed with pre-diabetes, monitoring your own blood sugar with a glucose meter periodically can be a valuable tool to help you track your blood sugar. A glucose meter can be purchased over the counter or prescribed by your doctor. All meters come with easy-to-follow instructions. The readings from the glucose meter will help you learn how different foods affect your blood glucose, or what times of day you may be high or low. You can decide how often to check your blood glucose, but two to three times weekly may be a good start.

Cholesterol and Triglycerides

The relationship between cholesterol and heart disease is well known. People with pre-diabetes or diabetes have more risk for heart disease; therefore, monitoring your cholesterol levels is an important part of your health plan. Knowing your total cholesterol is not sufficient to determine whether you are at risk. You also need to know how much of your total cholesterol represents good cholesterol (HDL, or high-density lipoprotein) or bad cholesterol (LDL, or low-density lipoprotein). Triglycerides, another type of fat found in the blood, are also associated with determining risk factors for heart disease. Below are recommended levels for cholesterol and triglyceride levels for individuals without diabetes or pre-diabetes. If you have pre-diabetes, your doctor may want to see readings even lower. The following list indicates normal laboratory values for cholesterol and triglycerides.

- Total cholesterol: Less than 200mg/dl
- LDL cholesterol: Less than 100mg/dl
- HDL cholesterol: Greater than 40mg/dl for men; greater than 50mg/dl for women
- Triglycerides: Less than 150mg/dl

LDL and HDL levels are much better predictors of heart disease risk than the total cholesterol. Although someone may have a normal total cholesterol reading, they can still be at increased risk if the LDL (bad) cholesterol is higher than recommended levels. If the results of your cholesterol or triglycerides are abnormal, you and your doctor will discuss these results. In addition to lab results, other risk factors such as gender, family history, smoking, weight, and blood pressure help determine the best course of treatment for you. For some individuals, healthy diet, modest weight loss, and a regular exercise plan may be enough to bring cholesterol and triglyceride levels in range. For others, the addition of cholesterol and/or triglyceride-lowering medications may be necessary.

ESSENTIAL

The lipid panel, which measures total cholesterol, HDL, LDL, and triglycerides, should be done at least annually. If your doctor has prescribed cholesterol- or triglyceride-lowering medications for you, a lipid panel, as well as other blood tests, may be required more often to monitor your body's response to the medication.

C-Reactive Protein (CRP)

C-reactive protein is a protein found in the blood that indicates the amount of inflammation in your body. Inflammation plays a role in pre-diabetes and diabetes. A high-sensitive C-reactive protein (hsCRP) test can identify low-grade inflammation that increases one's risk for developing heart disease, making this a useful test for people at high risk for heart disease. Elevated CRP levels can also be found in some people with pre-diabetes, diabetes, or who are overweight.

Blood Pressure

Just as the prevalence of pre-diabetes and diabetes is on the rise, having hypertension (high blood pressure) is on the rise as well. Being overweight and having a sedentary lifestyle are two key reasons for an increased prevalence of high blood pressure. Sodium intake in one's diet can be a cause of high blood pressure. The 2010 Dietary Guidelines for Americans recommends a reduction in daily sodium intake to less than 2,300 mg. For people who are fifty-one and older, and those of any age who are African American or have hypertension, diabetes, or chronic kidney disease, a further reduction to 1,500 mg daily is recommended. Although the recommendations for sodium intake have been reduced, many people consume much more sodium because they are using convenience, packaged, or processed foods often. Processed food accounts for a large percentage of the sodium Americans consume on a daily basis. A person who is salt sensitive may develop high blood pressure as a result of high sodium intake.

Blood pressure is the force of blood against the walls of arteries. The measurement is written one above the other, with the systolic number on top and the diastolic number on the bottom. Systolic blood pressure represents the force with which your heart pumps blood into the arteries. Diastolic blood pressure measures the pressure in the arteries when the heart is at rest, between heartbeats. High blood pressure needs to be treated because continued high pressure exerted on arteries can cause damage to the arteries or the heart.

The American College of Endocrinology (ACE) Task Force on the Prevention of Diabetes recommends a target blood pressure of 130/80 for persons with pre-diabetes. This is the same target for persons with diabetes.

About Metabolic Syndrome

Metabolic syndrome is a name used for a group of risk factors that, if present, increase your risk for having heart disease or other problems such as diabetes. Metabolic syndrome develops for many of the same reasons that pre-diabetes does. The treatment of metabolic syndrome is the same as for pre-diabetes. If you have a diagnosis of pre-diabetes, there may be a good chance that you have metabolic syndrome as well.

People who are overweight or obese and physically inactive are more likely to develop metabolic syndrome and insulin resistance. Having excess fat in the abdominal area and a large waist circumference increase the likelihood of insulin resistance.

Insulin resistance is a condition where the body is unable to use its own insulin properly. Insulin, a hormone made by the pancreas, helps the body to use glucose for energy. People with insulin resistance require and may produce more insulin to help glucose get into cells. A consistent overproduction of insulin, coupled with overeating, promotes weight gain. Eventually, the pancreas is no longer able to keep up with insulin demand and blood glucose begins to rise to the diabetic range.

ALERT

Metabolic syndrome means you have three or more conditions that together increase risk for heart disease, stroke, and diabetes. Specifically those conditions include: large waist circumference (more than 36 inches in women and 40 inches in men), blood pressure higher than 130/85 mmHg (millimeters of mercury), elevated triglyceride level and a low level of HDL cholesterol, and insulin resistance.

Family history and older age are other possible factors for metabolic syndrome. Obviously genetics and age cannot be controlled; however, weight, blood fats (blood lipids), blood pressure, and blood glucose are factors that you can have influence over.

Minority Populations at Risk

Certain groups of people are more affected by diabetes than others. African Americans and Hispanics are twice as likely to develop diabetes compared to Caucasians. This means that the prevalence of pre-diabetes in this group is also much higher. In the nation's health report, Healthy People 2010, it was reported that African Americans, Mexican Americans, and American Indians have had a very sharp rise in the number of people with type 2 diabetes over the last decade. Other minority groups affected by this trend include Native Hawaiians, Pacific Islanders, and Asian Americans.

FACT

The minority population in the United States has also grown over the last decade. This provides a partial explanation for why there are more people within minority groups who have diabetes. Changes in lifestyle and eating habits can provide another reason for the increase in diabetes or obesity. Traditional diets may be abandoned in favor of the Western diet. A change in eating pattern (adding highly processed or fast foods) can contribute to obesity or type 2 diabetes. Also, people may shift from a physically active lifestyle to one that is more sedentary.

Pregnancy and Pre-Diabetes

Pregnancy is a time of life when most women are very motivated to take very good care of themselves. They do this because they want the best possible outcome for their baby. For a woman with either pre-diabetes or gestational diabetes, good self-care is especially important and necessary to ensure a good outcome. Though there are differences between pre-diabetes and gestational diabetes, keep in mind that there is a definite connection between the two as well.

The diagnostic criteria for pre-diabetes usually starts with a fasting blood glucose between 100–125mg/dl on more than one occasion. If a woman has pre-diabetes at the onset of her pregnancy, her risk for developing gestational diabetes is increased.

Gestational Diabetes

Somewhere between 2–10 percent of all pregnant women develop gestational diabetes. It is more common in women who are older or overweight at the onset of their pregnancy, or if they had gestational diabetes in a prior pregnancy.

Gestational diabetes occurs when certain hormones from the placenta interfere with the normal action of the woman's insulin. Hormonal interference creates insulin resistance, and the woman's ability to use her own insulin to regulate blood sugar is greatly reduced. The pancreas, which produces insulin, cannot produce enough insulin to correct the insulin resistance, and high blood sugar levels are the result.

ALERT

Having diabetes during pregnancy can make a woman's pregnancy more complicated and require extra medical care. The potential problems that can occur with gestational or other types of diabetes include an increased chance of a miscarriage, cesarean section, or early delivery because of a larger size of the baby.

All pregnant women are screened for gestational diabetes between 24 and 28 weeks of the pregnancy. This is generally the time when gestational diabetes becomes evident. Women with glucose abnormalities such as pre-diabetes or a prior history of gestational diabetes may be screened earlier than this. The screening is done by measuring the mother's blood glucose one hour after she has consumed 50 grams of glucose. A blood glucose of 140 mg/dl or less is considered normal; if it is higher than that, further testing is done. When a second round of testing is performed, 100 grams of glucose is consumed and the blood glucose is measured at the fasting level, and every hour for the next two to three hours. Levels greater than the values below are indicative of gestational diabetes:

- Fasting: 92mg/dl
- One hour: 180mg/dl
- Two hours: 155mg/dl
- Three hours: 140mg/dl

Even under normal conditions, pregnancy is a stressful time for the body. In addition to the normal stresses of pregnancy, having pre-diabetes makes the risk for gestational diabetes that much greater. If you have pre-diabetes and are planning to become pregnant, be sure to get your pre-diabetes under control first. Discuss your plans for starting a family with your doctor, and follow recommendations for getting healthier before the pregnancy.

It may be a good idea to monitor your blood glucose a few times weekly, and have your doctor check your hemoglobin A1c to determine whether your pre-diabetes is well controlled.

I'm Pregnant and Have Pre-Diabetes . . . Now What?

If you are already pregnant and have pre-diabetes, it does not necessarily mean that you *will* develop gestational diabetes. Be proactive by improving your lifestyle habits right away. Learn about good nutrition and healthy eating habits. Make an appointment with a registered dietitian to review your current eating habits and discuss how you can make improvements. In most cases, the guidelines for healthy eating will be similar to those used for the woman with gestational diabetes. A diet that has moderate amounts of carbohydrates obtained mostly from whole grain foods, fresh fruit, and plenty of vegetables is usually recommended. Sweets, sugar, sweetened foods or beverages, and highly processed foods are kept to a minimum. Your dietitian can provide guidance about foods that are high in nutritional value yet low in calories to help you prevent excess weight gain during your pregnancy.

Keep weight gain under control throughout the pregnancy to minimize your chances of developing gestational diabetes! Follow your doctor's recommendations for the right amount of weight to gain during your pregnancy. Here are recommended guidelines for weight gain based on your weight at the start of the pregnancy:

- Underweight: 28–40 pounds
- Normal weight: 25–35 pounds
- Overweight: 15–25 pounds
- Obese: 11–20 pounds

Unless otherwise instructed by a doctor, all women, including those with pre-diabetes, should remain physically active throughout their pregnancy. Most women will be able to perform moderate-intensity exercise such as brisk walking. Aim for at least 150 minutes weekly. If you have not been physically active prior to your pregnancy, start slowly and gradually increase the amount of time you exercise. Avoid activities that put you at risk for abdominal injuries or a fall. Try to get routine, moderate exercise as long as you are able to throughout your pregnancy.

After Delivery

In most cases, gestational diabetes goes away after the baby is born. This is because the mother no longer has the hormones that interfered with insulin and raised her blood glucose. Women with a gestational diabetes history may be predisposed to type 2 diabetes at a later time in life.

The woman with pre-diabetes prior to or during her pregnancy may or may not have pre-diabetes afterward. The outcome in this situation is dependent upon certain variables such as amount of weight gain, diet, exercise, or level of glucose control during the pregnancy.

Whether you had to manage pre-diabetes or gestational diabetes during pregnancy, your decision to prevent type 2 diabetes requires a certain amount of vigilance after you have your baby. Maintain a healthy diet, get plenty of exercise, and prevent excess weight gain in the future. By staying on course with a healthy lifestyle, you will be taking the steps within your control to prevent type 2 diabetes in the future!

Polycystic Ovary Syndrome and Pre-Diabetes

Polycystic ovary syndrome (PCOS) affects approximately 5–10 percent of women in the United States. PCOS is defined as a grouping of reproductive health problems characterized by polycystic (many cysts) ovaries, irregular menstrual cycles, infertility, and obesity. It is the most common cause of irregular menstrual cycles and infertility. Most women with PCOS have *insulin resistance* and hyperinsulinism. Hyperinsulinism means that high amounts of insulin are routinely produced to combat the insulin resistance. Like metabolic syndrome, an overproduction of insulin triggers a cycle of easy weight gain.

Some women with PCOS also have metabolic syndrome and may have other symptoms such as acanthosis nigricans (dark skin patches), acne, facial hair, or loss of scalp hair. A woman with PCOS can go on to develop pre-diabetes or type 2 diabetes. Other conditions associated with PCOS may include obstructive sleep apnea, depression, or hypothyroidism.

QUESTION

Do women with PCOS have to follow a very low carbohydrate diet? Although there are no formal dietary guidelines for specific carbohydrate amounts in PCOS, it is known that refined carbohydrates are not beneficial. Many women with PCOS experience carbohydrate cravings triggered by the hyperinsulinism. Consuming refined carbohydrates can exacerbate this cycle. A moderate intake of carbohydrate is helpful in controlling cravings or hypoglycemia. Controlled portions of whole grains, fresh fruit, and vegetables are the recommended sources of carbohydrates. White flour products and other types of processed foods should be limited.

Lowering insulin levels and improving insulin sensitivity are the key strategies to managing PCOS. Without treatment of hyperinsulinism, weight gain and other metabolic abnormalities may occur. The treatment for PCOS is strikingly similar to treatment strategies used for pre-diabetes or metabolic syndrome. Weight loss, proper nutrition, and increased physical activity are considered essential components of treatment for PCOS. In some cases oral contraceptives to correct hormonal abnormalities or use of a medication such as Metformin (an insulin sensitizer used to treat diabetes) can improve symptoms associated with PCOS.

Children and Teens with Pre-Diabetes

With the medical advances over the decades, a gradual increase in the human life span has occurred for each successive generation. Now this trend may change, and for the first time in many years, today's children could have health issues or chronic disease at a much earlier age in life compared to their parents or grandparents. Earlier onset of chronic disease could mean a decline in the life expectancies of the younger generation. The increased incidence of obesity and pre-diabetes in our children plays a major role in this unfortunate development.

Thirty years ago it was uncommon to see a child with pre-diabetes. Today healthcare practitioners not only see children and adolescents with pre-diabetes, they diagnose and treat type 2 diabetes in this very population. Type

2 diabetes was once regarded as an adult-onset form of diabetes, and not a form of diabetes that affected children or adolescents. According to data from the National Diabetes Fact Sheet 2007, there were approximately two million adolescents (or one in six overweight adolescents) with pre-diabetes.

Children and teens are more at risk for pre-diabetes or diabetes if:

- They are overweight or obese
- They have a parent, sibling, or other close relative with type 2 diabetes
- They do not get enough physical activity
- They are American Indian, African American, Asian American, or Hispanic/Latino

Although it is not possible to change one's genetic or family background, maintaining a healthy weight and staying active are two areas that you and your child have control of. It is much easier to correct a small problem before it becomes a big problem. If your child is gaining extra weight, take steps to reverse the situation as soon as possible. Even if your child displays no signs of pre-diabetes, a healthy weight and adequate activity are vitally important in the prevention of this condition.

The Role of BMI

For many years doctors relied on height and weight measurements to assess a child's growth pattern. Height and weight are usually reviewed during the annual health checkup. Another way to determine whether a child is at a healthy weight is to calculate his or her body mass index (BMI). BMI is a calculation that uses height and weight to estimate how much body fat a person has. The BMI calculation for children is not interpreted in the same way as normal BMI ranges for adults. Although the mathematical method used to determine the BMI is the same, a child's BMI is compared to typical values for other children of the same age and gender. For children aged two through twenty, a BMI that is less than the fifth percentile is considered underweight and above the ninety-fifth percentile is considered obese. A BMI between the eighty-fifth and ninety-fifth percentile is classified as overweight.

During your child's next checkup at the doctor's office, learn what his BMI and BMI percentile are. You can also determine this on your own by using the *Kid's Health BMI Calculator* found at this website: *http:// kidshealth.org/parent/growth/growth/bmi_charts.html*. To use this calculator, you will need to enter height, weight, age, and gender.

If your child's BMI indicates an overweight status, keep in mind that he is still growing. In some cases an overweight child may grow out of the overweight category as he gets taller and older. Because of growth, it is important to check your child's BMI routinely, to see whether it has improved or gotten worse.

When children or teens remain in the overweight or obese category, there should be screening for pre-diabetes and diabetes. Screening is especially important when additional risk factors such as family history of diabetes or ethnic specificity are present.

The laboratory tests to screen children and teens for pre-diabetes or diabetes are the same as those used for adults. A fasting blood glucose (after an overnight fast) should be under 100mg/dl. Some doctors prefer to use the glucose challenge when screening children. Based on the child's body weight, a specific number of grams of glucose are consumed, and the blood glucose is checked two hours later. A healthy child will have a result of less than 140mg/dl after two hours. If the hemoglobin A1c test is used, a result of 6.0–6.5 percent is indicative of pre-diabetes.

What to Do If Your Child Has Pre-Diabetes

As upsetting as the news may be, your child's diagnosis of pre-diabetes is very treatable and, with the right plan in place, reversible. Put your child's mind at ease by letting him know that you are going to be there to help. It is important for your child to understand that certain changes in eating and exercise habits are necessary to prevent future health problems. At the same time, you need to present this information in a way so that your child does not become fearful or excessively worried about his condition.

To have success with lifestyle improvements, change really has to become a family affair. In other words, you and other family members must be supportive and participate in the lifestyle changes that need to take place. Don't expect your child or teen to "go it alone," while others in the household continue to have poor eating or lifestyle habits. If your child feels as though he has been singled out, you will very likely meet with resistance.

It is important to get your child actively engaged and involved in the process of change. He will be more likely to "buy in" to new changes when he is involved in some of the decision making, and not just told what to do! For example, let your child decide what healthy after-school snack he would like to eat, instead of selecting items for him. Although grocery shopping takes more time with children present, it is worthwhile to take your child along from time to time. Shopping trips can help your child see and learn about different food options, as well as provide an opportunity to choose healthy foods.

As a parent, your most important job is to set a good example, and having a healthy lifestyle is no exception. Early on, children learn by example and copy their parents' behavior. For example, parents who don't eat vegetables can hardly expect their child to start eating them willingly on their own! Model healthy lifestyle and eating habits yourself, and you will have a much better chance of having your child follow your good example.

Here are some things that families can do together that will not only help the child or teen with pre-diabetes but also improves everyone's state of health:

- Make less frequent visits to fast food restaurants or restaurants that offer all-you-can-eat buffets
- Limit the amount of sweetened or salty snack foods that are brought into the home
- Switch out soda and juice boxes for bottled water or low-fat milk
- Have plenty of healthy snack items available at home such as fresh fruit, low-fat yogurt, or raw vegetables
- Get more physical activity: This means more than simply telling a child to exercise! A walk or short bike ride together are good examples of how to get everyone at home moving.
- Cut down on TV or video-game time every day. Put a limit of one to two hours for TV or video-game time a day. That is more than enough time for passive activities.

QUESTION

My child has pre-diabetes. Does this mean he is going to develop type 2 diabetes?
Progressing from pre-diabetes to type 2 diabetes is not inevitable! When positive lifestyle changes are made, pre-diabetes may be reversible. Your child needs to know that there are many choices he can make to stay healthy. Even if he does develop diabetes, he needs to know that children with diabetes thrive and can remain healthy throughout their lives. In fact, some children with diabetes are healthier than those who don't have it, because they are following a healthy plan of diet and exercise!

Some Things to Keep in Mind

By now you understand the importance of helping your child start a healthy eating and exercise program sooner rather than later. Most of us (your child included) have established eating habits that may be hard to break. Working little by little on ways to eat healthier takes time and patience. The same goes for taking on more activity or exercise. A child who prefers passive activities such as watching television will need time to get used to getting physical activity every day. Old habits are hard to break and without daily practice of new habits, it's easy to get off track or revert to old behavior. Success usually comes by starting with small changes and mastering a new behavior before taking on more challenges. One or two positive changes at a time is realistic and prevents your child from becoming overwhelmed. Do not get discouraged if your child or teen does not immediately change all of her poor health habits. Even adults struggle with lifestyle change and have to try over and over again. Your job is to encourage your child to keep trying!

Ultimately, children and teens want to be accepted by their peers. At some level they understand that being overweight or having health problems can make it more difficult to develop friendships, play in sports, or participate in social activities. Healthy habits will help your child gain more confidence and control over his own well-being, and this can have a positive effect on other areas of his life!

CHAPTER 3

Your Action Plan for Pre-Diabetes

By now you understand the potential consequences of untreated pre-diabetes. It is important to develop an action plan. Your action plan will help you make lifestyle changes gradually that will be implemented on a day-to-day basis. Have specific, tangible goals to work on. Generally, no more than two or three specific goals should be worked on at one time. This strategy prevents you from getting overwhelmed and allows you to master a goal before moving on to something else. Building in a small reward system for goals achieved can be a powerful way to keep you motivated. Rewards such as buying a new CD or book, going to a movie, or spending leisure time on a favorite hobby are examples of ways to celebrate progress.

Halting the Progression of Pre-Diabetes

Halting the progression of pre-diabetes is extremely important and necessary to restore good health. With pre-diabetes, there is still a chance for you to reverse the progression and prevent the onset of type 2 diabetes. Even if you develop diabetes eventually at a later time, slowing down the progression will result in fewer complications. Without taking action, progression to full-blown type 2 diabetes is a likely possibility.

There are three essential components to your action plan. First, most people with pre-diabetes will need to lose weight. Although you may know what it takes to lose weight, being consistent and keeping weight off is much more of a challenge than actually losing the weight. Second, you will need to work on gradual behavioral changes such as eating out less often or focusing on portion control. Third, you will need to begin and maintain a routine exercise plan that is right for you.

Your Weight's Influence on Pre-Diabetes

Your weight may be only one of several causes for pre-diabetes; however, it is one factor that can you can control. Body Mass Index (BMI) is the primary way healthcare practitioners determine whether you are at a healthy weight, overweight, or obese. It is important to know your BMI. As you begin to lose weight, you can adjust and track your BMI.

BMI can be determined using a special BMI chart. If you do not have a chart available, you can calculate your BMI in the following way:

1. Multiply your weight in pounds by 703.
2. Divide the result by your height in inches.
3. Divide this result by your height in inches again, and this will be your BMI.

A BMI of 18.5 to 24.9 is considered normal weight.
A BMI of 25 to 29.9 is considered overweight.
A BMI of 30 or greater is considered obese.
If you prefer to use a BMI calculator, go to *http://nhlbisupport.com/bmi*. There are many rewards that come with weight loss. Studies have shown that weight loss of as little as ten to twenty pounds can prevent or delay progression

to diabetes. Even weight loss of a just few pounds will provide health benefits right away. Once you begin losing weight, insulin resistance will be reduced and insulin sensitivity will increase. This means that your blood glucose levels will be lower long before you reach your weight goal. Over time, weight loss can help reduce blood lipid (cholesterol and triglyceride) levels and lower blood pressure. For some, lower lipid levels or blood pressure can reduce the need for medication. An overall reduction in weight reduces the chances of having a heart attack, stroke, gallbladder disease, bone or joint problems, and certain types of cancer. Problems related to poor quality sleep, sleep apnea, and other breathing problems are known to improve with weight loss.

ESSENTIAL

Expecting that you will lose weight quickly is not realistic or long lasting. Losing one half to one pound a week over a period of time will go much further in helping you achieve results. Instead of focusing on a specific weight number on the scale, use positive observations to stay on track. Clothing that fits better or an increased energy level are good ways to gauge your progress. Whatever amount of weight you lose will be of benefit.

The point in time when modest weight loss is most likely to improve your health is when you have pre-diabetes or are in the very early stages of diabetes. Over time, persons with type 2 diabetes lose the ability to make adequate amounts of insulin. When this happens, weight loss and exercise alone are not enough to control blood glucose. Medications to lower blood glucose become a necessary part of treatment. Knowing that you may be able to avoid the need for medication is a good motivator for losing weight and keeping it off.

Facing Your Food Problems

You probably can identify certain food choices you make that need to be changed because of the ill effect they have on your health and weight. For some people it's salty snack foods, for others it may be ice cream or bakery items. Now is a good time to identify your problem foods and work on ways to reduce your exposure to them.

It's important to learn how to make your food environment safe and keep it as free as possible from foods that can cause problem eating and extra calories. Start by reviewing the foods you routinely buy at the grocery store. Are these foods helping you reach your goals or are they self-sabotaging? What kinds of foods are in the cupboards or freezer? Many people have a hard time cleaning up their food environment because of other people living in the household. Keeping salty snacks or ice cream in the house because "the kids want them" is not likely to help you stay on track. Remember that healthy eating should be for everyone, and having problem foods around the house makes it difficult for anyone to resist eating those foods. Discuss your food problems with your family and come to some agreements regarding how often and how much of these foods should be allowed in the household. Help your family understand that if tempting, high-calorie foods are in the house all of the time, you are not going to be able to ignore them!

Foods that are sweet or salty taste good and temporarily make you feel good. The problem is, the immediate satisfaction you get from these foods is hard to pass up, and in no time at all you are back for more. Relying on will-power to stop you from eating irresistible foods will not work if faced with these food choices every day. In fact, willpower should not be one of your ongoing strategies to improve your eating habits. Make your food environment safer by keeping healthier food and snack alternatives available at all times. Remove your problem foods from the house on a regular basis and you will begin to move away from consuming these foods.

Of course, it is difficult (and for most, pretty impossible) to never eat the foods you love. If you decide never to eat a particular food, you may become obsessed with it and end up overeating it when given the opportunity. Instead, give yourself permission to have the food during a special occasion or celebration. Find a way to balance the problem food in a healthy way by not restricting but rather reserving it for a certain time when you are free to really enjoy it. Lifelong healthy eating is about choice and finding a way to balance all the foods that you enjoy.

When you go grocery shopping, be sure to purchase a few healthy snack items. Many people find that if they have healthy snacks available, it becomes easier to use them in the absence of the high-calorie snacks. Availability of healthy food takes away the impulsiveness of poor food decisions.

FACT

Having one or two snacks during the day is a good way to keep your blood glucose stable and take the edge off your hunger. By using low-calorie snacks between meals, you can feel satisfied until your next meal. Try to keep your snacks in the range of 100–200 calories.

Here are a few examples of low-calorie snacks to have available in your safe food environment:

- Carrot sticks or sliced peppers with 2 tablespoons hummus for dipping
- Low-fat mozzarella cheese stick and a small apple
- 1 tablespoon peanut butter on 4 whole-grain crackers
- 6 ounces light or plain yogurt with ¼ cup berries
- 10–12 nuts and a small piece of fruit of your choice

Get Moving (Every Day!)

Exercise has to be part of your action plan for halting pre-diabetes. The role of exercise cannot be underestimated or lacking from your overall plan. Before starting an exercise program, decide what you can do and how to keep it as simple as possible. Too often, people become overenthusiastic at first, overdo it, and then burn out. Once this happens, they may not resume exercise at all. Start with one easy goal and master it for a few weeks before moving on to something else.

For some, the most difficult part of exercise is figuring out when they can fit it into their busy days. If this is you, try keeping a log of your daily activities for several days, then examine where there may be a small block of time to work in some exercise.

CHAPTER 4

Exercise:
Essential for Your Success

Being more active is an important part of your pre-diabetes plan. Regular activity and exercise will improve your blood glucose levels. Lower blood glucose levels are achieved when the glucose in your blood is used for energy during and after exercise. Muscle cells become more sensitive to insulin, allowing for better storage and usage of glucose for energy. Cells in the liver also become more sensitive to insulin, and this helps prevent the liver from producing too much glucose. In essence, insulin resistance improves with regular exercise, and gradually blood glucose levels go down. Routine exercise is vital to the process of stopping pre-diabetes from progressing to diabetes, and improving your general health.

How Do You Get Started?

When you first learned about having pre-diabetes, your doctor probably encouraged you to begin exercising. If this was not initially discussed, you should talk to your doctor to make sure that exercise is appropriate for you. In most cases, your doctor will support your desire to start an exercise plan. If you have other health issues in addition to pre-diabetes, you and your doctor will want to discuss the best types of exercise for you. Be realistic when choosing exercises for yourself. Once your doctor has given you the okay to start, it's time to consider the variables that will help you choose the right type of exercise:

- Consider your physical ability to perform certain activities and choose activities that you can do. Some exercises may be too difficult or strenuous for your current level of fitness.
- Include activities you enjoy or those already performed on a regular basis. Going for a walk, gardening, or vacuuming are all activities that can easily help get you moving and be part of your daily routine.
- Think about how much time you have. An ambitious exercise plan that involves too much time will quickly be abandoned if you lack the time. If you have not exercised recently, ease into a program that includes short periods of time to start with.
- Consider the resources available to you. If you do not have access to a gym, exercise equipment, or a pool, then a simple walking plan may be your best bet.

ALERT

Resist the temptation to purchase home exercise equipment until you have tried it out and are reasonably sure that you will use it. Many types of home equipment end up at garage sales or just taking up space because the owner stopped using the equipment after a short period of time. If you are considering buying home exercise equipment, try it out first in the store, at a gym, or a friend's house before purchasing it. Make sure you like the activity enough that you will want to do it often!

When you make plans for exercise and activity, it is important to be honest about your likelihood to maintain the plan. Make sure to have activities that you will enjoy, or do not mind doing. Would you prefer to exercise alone or with the company of a friend or spouse? Will your activity involve being outdoors or indoors? Can you perform the activity outdoors year-round or will you need to find an alternate indoor activity for part of the year? Try to work out any barriers ahead of time that could get in the way of your exercise plan.

Making Time for Exercise

Your exercise routine should be planned to fit naturally into your daily schedule. Look at your daily routine, then decide where you can realistically fit in some time for activity. Short periods of time (ten to thirty minutes) will probably work much better than trying to carve out an hour for daily activity. Start out with small amounts of time one or more times a day. You will likely have more success getting in activity this way. Here are a few examples of how you can slip in a little bit of activity every day without making huge demands on your schedule:

- Find opportunities to walk by arriving at your destination early, parking further away, then walking for ten minutes.
- During the workday, get up from your desk to walk around every hour. Take the stairs whenever you can and do this several times during the day.
- Go for a ten-minute walk after lunch or dinner.
- Spend ten minutes at the beginning and end of each day doing a few stretching exercises.
- Remember that many routine household activities such as cleaning, vacuuming, carrying groceries, gardening, and yard work are all forms of physical activity. Include this type of activity in your daily routine.

Get Walking!

For most people walking is a good place to begin because it is easy and requires no special equipment other than a pair of good walking shoes or sneakers. If you choose to walk and have not exercised in a long time, you may need to begin by walking at a moderate pace. Walking about three times a week for a period of ten to fifteen minutes can help ease you into a routine. As you become stronger and gain more endurance, gradually increase your walking time by five minutes every one to two weeks, until you are able to walk for a full thirty minutes. Once you are comfortable walking for thirty minutes, increase your frequency to four or five times weekly, and gradually pick up the pace to a brisk walk. Brisk walking is considered an aerobic exercise, which means oxygen is used. Aerobic exercise increases your heart rate and burns calories. Walking in this manner is considered an effective type of exercise for weight loss. In addition to brisk walking, running, jogging, dancing, cycling, and swimming are examples of aerobic exercise. Generally, the more vigorous the aerobic exercise and the longer time you do it, the more benefits you will gain.

An excellent way to stay motivated and track your progress with walking is to use a pedometer. A pedometer is an inexpensive small device that counts the number of steps you take in the course of the day. A pedometer is usually clipped to a belt or waistband, and if worn from the beginning to the end of your day, will count each step that you take. You can determine your daily step total by wearing the pedometer for three consecutive full days, then dividing the step total by three. Once you know the average steps you take per day, you can set small goals for yourself to increase the total number of steps you take every day.

QUESTION

What is the best time of day to exercise?
As long as you exercise, the time of day you actually do the exercise is the best time! Busy and demanding schedules often get in the way of good intentions. If your schedule is particularly demanding, try making an appointment on your schedule for your exercise time. Remember that any time spent exercising is better than no time!

To learn more about walking and using a pedometer, you may want to visit the site *www.shapeup.org/shape/resources/10ksteps.html*. The Shape Up America website can help you learn more about walking as a means to lose weight and improve fitness. The site provides encouragement and guidance for reaching 10,000 steps a day!

No Exercise = Little to No Results

If you really want to stop pre-diabetes in its tracks, it is important to understand just how important it is to initiate a plan for physical activity. Many people just focus on changing their eating habits. While this is very important, the lack of exercise could prevent you from reaching your goals. Cutting down on food will not be enough to help you lose weight and maintain a lower weight. Physical activity is a key component to your pre-diabetes plan and must be included at whatever level you are able to accommodate. Exercise is often left out because of perceived barriers that keep someone from becoming more active. If you are someone who never seems able to find the time or energy for exercise, begin to take a serious look at what the barriers are. Once you identify what is getting in your way, plan strategies to help you go around those barriers. Keep your strategies simple and real. Writing down and implementing your strategy is a good way to help you make permanent changes.

ESSENTIAL

Consistent exercise provides many rewards for everyone and especially for people with pre-diabetes. Preventing or delaying diabetes is at the top of the list, but you will also enjoy lower blood glucose and A1c levels, lower blood pressure, lower lipid levels, a more toned body, reduced stress, and better sleep!

Slow and Steady Wins the Race

Once you have had success with starting and maintaining your exercise, branch out and find new ways to get exercise and keep it interesting. Varying the routine helps to keep you from getting bored, and it challenges your body in different ways. An exercise plan of walking can be augmented by including strength training and stretching. Strength training helps to build muscle. Increasing muscle mass reduces insulin resistance and helps to lower blood glucose. Examples of strength training include lifting weights, push-ups, squats, lunges, and pull-ups. If you include strength training, be sure to allow at least forty-eight hours between sessions so your muscles are able to rest and recover. For most people, short strength-training sessions two to three times weekly will provide added benefit. Stretching is another worthy addition to a well-rounded exercise plan because it helps to increase flexibility and prevent injury. Stretch slowly, without bouncing, and only stretch as far as you can without causing any pain. A few minutes of stretching at the beginning and end of an exercise session can make exercise easier and reduce the possibility of injury.

Your exercise program should be one that you can maintain for life. Make sensible decisions about what you can and will change to increase your activity level. You may realize some of the benefits of exercise early on, but long-lasting results come about with consistency. Think of your exercise program as a work in progress that you are constantly improving and finding new ways to derive health benefits and enjoyment from. Slow, steady progress will help you achieve your goals, and you will realize how worthwhile your efforts have been.

How to Help Your Children Become More Active

For children and teens physical activity is an essential part of a healthy lifestyle, and helps prevent many chronic diseases. Unfortunately, today's children and teens are much less physically active than their parents were. Bicycle riding and jumping rope have been replaced with computer games and phone texting. To get your child's cooperation, help him understand *why* exercise has to become a regular part of his life. Be positive and emphasize the benefits such as:

- Exercise is essential for keeping a body healthy and strong and for building lean muscle.
- Individuals who are active and fit sustain far fewer illnesses or injuries.
- Physical activity is necessary for maintenance of normal weight.

- Exercise can help with better sleep and is effective for reducing stress.
- Perhaps the most important reason for a child with pre-diabetes to get exercise: It helps to bring blood glucose back to normal!

Fitting Activity Into Every Day

There are plenty of things your child or teen can do to become active every day. Talk with your child about what type of activities he thinks might be fun or interesting to try. If other family members or friends participate in the activity too, he will be more willing to go along. It is more fun to be active with others. Think about programs offered at the YMCA, YWCA, or other community groups that offer physical activity. Offer to go for a walk or bike ride with your child after dinner. Perhaps trying a new activity such as skateboarding, bowling, or an after-school activity might be appealing.

QUESTION

How much exercise does my child need?
Children and teens need about sixty minutes of exercise at least five days a week. If this seems like a lot of time, consider the amount of time they may be spending watching TV or using the computer, video games, or cell phones. For most children, it adds up to almost seven and a half hours a day!

Even walking to and from school is a great way to start getting more active! Get an inexpensive pedometer for your child, so he can count daily activity steps, and work toward achieving 10,000 steps a day. Some studies suggest that 10,000 steps a day is about the right amount of steps to be considered exercise. When a pedometer is used to figure out how many steps are taken every day, you may be surprised to learn that your child is not moving nearly enough.

How Much Is Enough?

It is perfectly okay to break up sixty minutes of physical activity into shorter intervals during the day. For example, thirty minutes of gym class at school could be complemented with thirty minutes of play outside after school. If your child has not been active and seems to tire quickly, encourage him or her to start out slowly (less time) and keep at it! Fifteen minutes twice a day may be enough for a start.

Remember that being active can take on many different forms and it does not have to be formal exercise. If your child gets involved with routine activities around the home, this can serve as a great way to get exercise and possibly earn an allowance or reward from you! Whether it's mowing the lawn, raking leaves, or washing the car, it all counts as physical activity!

The Alliance for a Healthier Generation (*www.healthiergeneration.org*) and Let's Move (*www.letsmove.gov*) are helpful websites offering practical ideas to parents and children working toward healthy lifestyle behaviors.

CHAPTER 5

What Can You Eat?

You may think that having pre-diabetes means you will have to give up everything you like to eat, especially carbohydrates. Nothing could be further from the truth! With the help and advice of a registered dietitian, you can adapt healthy eating habits that fit into your lifestyle. Realize that you won't be able to change your eating habits overnight. It is much easier to adopt the approach of taking small steps every day. Over time, you can make significant changes toward improving your health and reaching near-normal blood glucose levels consistently.

Keep It Simple to Start

Think of changes in your eating habits as goals rather than inflexible rules and regulations. Start by making an honest review of your current eating habits and list the things you would like to change or improve. If you brainstorm a bit, you will be able to come up with quite a few positive changes that you could make. Decide exactly what you need to do in order to bring about change, and then select one or two changes to work on at a time. Here are a few ideas to help you start this process:

- **Eat meals at regular intervals.** Resolve not to skip meals or go for long periods of time without eating.
- **Include nutritious snacks in your daily eating plan.** Fruits and vegetables are good choices.
- **Experiment with whole grains, vegetables, or fruits you have never tried before.** Check out the produce or whole foods section of your grocery store to see what's new.
- **Start reducing your portion sizes.** Cut back by 25–30 percent to get used to eating less.
- **Drink plenty of water every day.** Most adults need at least 48–64 ounces daily.

Once you've mastered a change, it's time to move on to something new. Some changes will be easy, and others will be difficult or take more time. Start by making easier changes first before tackling something that would be very difficult for you. This will help build your confidence.

Balance and Moderation Are Key

Everyone has the same nutritional needs regardless of whether or not they have pre-diabetes. You may be surprised to learn that your eating plan will have the same foods that everyone else eats (or should be eating!), and buying all sorts of specialty or diet foods is usually unnecessary. You may wish to use an artificial sweetener of your choice or certain sugar-free food items to add variety; however, this is not essential. You will not have to prepare one meal for yourself and something different for the rest of your family. As you look over the recipes in this book, you may want to try a few specialty items, but the recipes in general use ingredients that everyone can eat. To put it simply, a meal plan for managing pre-diabetes is a plan that most people can follow for good health.

ESSENTIAL

Eating a balanced diet that includes foods from all of the essential food groups generally meets the nutrition needs of most adults. Some individuals have other health issues in addition to pre-diabetes, and this may affect specific nutritional requirements. Discuss all of your health issues with your doctor and registered dietitian to determine whether you should take vitamin and mineral supplements to help meet specific nutritional needs.

Carbohydrates and Pre-Diabetes: Facts You Should Know

Carbohydrates serve as the body's primary energy source. Simple carbohydrates include sugars, sweets, juices, and fruits. Complex carbohydrates include all types of grain products and starchy vegetables such as potatoes and corn. Recommendations for a healthy diet and pre-diabetes suggest that most carbohydrates come from the complex carbohydrates rather than simple sugars. Complex carbohydrates found in whole-grain foods provide better nutritional value and are an important source of vitamins, minerals, and fiber. Fruit contains natural simple sugars, and they are also sources of vitamins, minerals, and fiber. To get the most fiber from fruit choose fresh or frozen, unsweetened fruit instead of fruit juice.

Having pre-diabetes or diabetes does not mean you must cut out all carbohydrates from your diet. You will be happy to learn that there are many carbohydrate food choices that you can include in your plan! Choose carbohydrates that have good nutritional value and maintain an appropriate portion size.

Proteins: Your Building Blocks to Good Health

Proteins are the building blocks of the body and are used for growth, building, and repair. Animal proteins such as meat, fish, eggs, and milk contain all nine essential amino acids. When all essential amino acids are present in food, it is called a complete protein.

Vegetable proteins are found in nuts, seeds, vegetables, whole grains, and legumes. All vegetable proteins, with the exception of soy, are considered incomplete proteins because one or more of the essential amino acids are missing. Even though a vegetable protein is considered incomplete, it is not considered less nutritious than a complete protein. Incomplete proteins simply need to be combined with other foods to provide the full complement of the nine essential amino acids. For example, combining rice (a grain) with beans (a legume) provides all of the essential amino acids. Combining grains, beans, nuts, vegetables, or seeds in various ways can provide a complete protein.

QUESTION

What are whole grains?
The FDA has defined whole grains as "the intact, ground, cracked, or flaked fruit of the grains whose principal components—the starchy endosperm, germ, and bran—are present in the same relative proportions as they exist in the intact grain." In other words, no part of the grain has been removed during processing and so you are getting all of the parts of a grain.

Fats: Polys, Monos, Saturated, and Trans

All fats, regardless of the type, have a significant amount of calories. Therefore, moderation of any fat is your best choice. Every gram of fat contains 9 calories.

Monounsaturated fat should make up most of the fat you consume. This type of fat is found in certain plant foods such as walnuts, canola oil, peanut oil, and olive oil. Monounsaturated fat does not raise blood cholesterol and may actually help reduce blood cholesterol levels if it replaces saturated fat in the diet.

Polyunsaturated fat should be used in moderation, and less often than monounsaturated fat. This fat come mostly from vegetable sources such as corn oil, sunflower oil, and some types of margarine.

Saturated fat should be used the least. This type of fat is typically found in foods made from animal sources such as meat, butter, cheese, or cream.

Baked goods such as cakes or pastries may be high in saturated fat if lard, palm, or coconut oils are used. Excessive intake of saturated fat can increase blood cholesterol levels.

Trans fat is the result of a food manufacturing process called hydrogenation. This process converts a liquid vegetable oil to a solid fat to make shortenings and solid (stick) types of margarine.

Foods containing omega-3 fatty acids are encouraged. Omega-3 plays an important role in the maintenance of immune function, brain development, and reproduction. There is considerable evidence to suggest that omega-3 fatty acids can have a positive effect on certain conditions due to their anti-inflammatory properties. Omega-3 fatty acids are found in soy oil, green leafy vegetables, walnuts, flax seed, and most notably, oily fish such as salmon, sardines, and mackerel.

ALERT

Check food labels and ingredients to avoid trans fat as much as possible. This form of fat can raise LDL (bad) cholesterol and increase your risk for heart disease. Trans fat can be found in vegetable shortenings, solid margarines, certain crackers, cookies, and other foods made with partially hydrogenated oils.

Cholesterol

Cholesterol is a waxy substance found in all body cells. It is part of some hormones and essential for fat digestion. The liver manufactures much of the cholesterol your body needs, but cholesterol is also obtained from the foods you eat. Cholesterol is found in animal foods such as meat, eggs, butter, and whole dairy products. Too much cholesterol in the blood can increase your risk for heart disease. People with pre-diabetes or diabetes have more risk for heart disease and should have their blood cholesterol checked routinely. Limit consumption of fatty meats, butter, and whole dairy foods such as whole milk or whole milk cheeses. Your doctor or registered dietitian may provide you with more specific recommendations for cholesterol control.

Sodium

Sodium is a mineral that does not affect blood sugar, but it can alter your blood pressure. Controlling blood pressure is yet another important aspect of managing pre-diabetes and preventing heart disease. The current Dietary Guidelines for Americans recommends a sodium intake for healthy adults of no more than 2,300 mg of sodium per day. Achieving this goal is particularly challenging for individuals who rely on packaged or processed foods as a large part of their diet. By reducing consumption of processed foods and including more whole foods, daily sodium consumption can be reduced. Here are some tips for reducing sodium:

- Leave out or reduce the amount of salt in standard recipes by 25–50 percent.
- Use commercial herb blends (or make your own using the recipes in Chapter 17 of this book) to season food instead of using salt.
- Limit intake of highly processed foods such as boxed mixes, instant foods, or processed meats.
- Make more soups, stews, casseroles, or side dishes from scratch.
- Watch your use of the salt shaker when cooking or at the table.

About Carbs, Fiber, and Whole Grains

There are two types of fiber found in foods: soluble and insoluble. It's important to include foods containing both types of fiber in your daily eating plan.

Soluble fiber dissolves or swells when it's put into water. This type of fiber helps keep blood sugar levels stable by slowing down the rate of glucose absorption into the bloodstream. Soluble fiber, when consumed in adequate amounts, can help lower blood cholesterol levels as well. Beans, fruit, barley, and oats are especially good sources of soluble fiber.

Insoluble fiber does not dissolve in water. In the body, it is not readily broken down by bacteria in the intestinal tract and this type of fiber passes through the body. Insoluble fiber is essential for preventing constipation and diverticulosis by helping to maintain regularity. Vegetables, whole-grain foods, and fruit are all good sources of insoluble fiber.

Getting More Fiber Every Day

Although all types of grains are sources of complex carbohydrates, those that have not been refined are better for you. Whole grains have more fiber and minerals. Whole grains have not had the bran layer and germ removed during the milling process; therefore, the fiber as well as vitamins and minerals are preserved. In addition, fiber helps to slow down the absorption of glucose into the bloodstream, which is important in the management of blood glucose. Refined grains such as white flour or white rice have the bran and germ removed, making them much lower in fiber, and vitamins and minerals are also lost during this process. Refined grains must have certain vitamins and minerals added back into the product after processing. Adding back nutrients to a processed food is called enrichment. When a label lists "enriched flour" as an ingredient, odds are it has been refined and may not be very high in fiber. Eating refined grains instead of whole grains makes it difficult to achieve adequate amounts of fiber each day. Whenever you can, choose whole grains over refined grains. The recommendation for daily fiber intake is 25–30 grams per day, which is about twice the amount found in the typical American diet.

FACT

Words like multigrain, seven-grain, or stone-ground do not necessarily mean a product is whole grain. If a whole-grain ingredient is not listed as the first ingredient, the item may contain only a small portion of whole grains. One way to find a whole-grain product is to look for the Whole Grains Council stamp of approval, which has two different logos used to label foods containing whole grains. The logo that reads "100% Whole Grain" indicates that the food has only whole grains and at least 16g per serving. The other label indicates only that a product contains whole grains.

Great Ways to Get More Whole Grains

The best way to get more whole grains in your meals is to substitute whole-grain foods for refined products. Here are some tips:

- When a recipe calls for white flour (all-purpose), experiment by replacing some of the flour with a whole-grain variety.
- Use a whole grain as a side dish or mix it with vegetables, lentils, or beans.
- Every week try one "new" grain that you have not used before. Quinoa, brown rice, bulgur, or kasha may be unfamiliar to you, but are as easy to prepare as white rice.
- Add whole grains to soups, salads, or casseroles instead of white rice or pasta.
- Try a cooked whole grain as a hot breakfast cereal.
- If you are not used to bran or other high-fiber cereals, try mixing them with equal amounts of your regular cereal.
- Switch to whole-grain crackers instead of saltines or other white-flour snack crackers.
- Use oatmeal in place of bread crumbs in items such as meatloaf or meatballs.
- Gradually start replacing the refined grains in your kitchen cabinets with whole-grain foods.

Gluten-Free Whole Grains

Consider adding gluten-free whole grains to your eating plan, even if you don't have celiac disease or a gluten/wheat intolerance. Many gluten-free whole grains are a wonderful source of fiber and essential nutrients. Gluten-free whole grains are available in their whole form or as flours. A few examples to consider include amaranth, buckwheat, teff, sorghum, quinoa, and montina (Indian rice grass).

CHAPTER 6

Translating Nutrition Into Real Meals

Knowing about good nutrition or the types of foods that you should eat when you have pre-diabetes is not enough. Translating what you know into an actual plan with healthy meals is very important! In this chapter you will learn more about using nutrition information to make wiser food choices whether you are shopping for food, dining out, or preparing your own meals.

Reading Food Labels

The Nutrition Facts found on food labels contain plenty of information, but unless you understand how to read the labels, you may be presented with information that doesn't mean very much to you.

Understanding Terms on Food Labels

- **Serving size:** Each label must identify the size of a serving. The nutritional information listed on a label is based on one serving of the food. Note that the serving listed on a package may not be the same as the size of your serving.
- **Amount per serving:** Each package identifies the quantities of nutrients and food constituents from one serving. From this information, you can find the caloric value of the food, in addition to the amount of fat (saturated or trans fat), cholesterol, sodium, carbohydrates, and protein per serving.
- **Percent daily value:** This indicates how much of a specific nutrient a serving of food contains in comparison to an average 2,000-calorie diet.
- **Ingredient list:** A listing of the ingredients in a food in descending order of predominance and weight.

Compare Carbohydrate Grams to Grams of Sugar

There are several parts to the carbohydrate section of the nutrition label. *Total Carbohydrate* represents the amount of carbohydrate grams found in a food. If the amount of carbohydrate grams is very high, you may decide whether or not it will fit into your eating plan. Beneath the Total Carbohydrate line are other listings: Fiber, Sugars, and sometimes, Sugar Alcohols. These values are all part of Total Carbohydrate.

ESSENTIAL

By comparing the calories from fat to the total calories in a food, you can identify foods that have lots of hidden fat. A typical hot dog has 110 total calories and 90 calories from fat. This means that 82 percent of the calories in the hot dog come from fat! Making this determination before buying a food can help you make much healthier choices. Look for foods that have 30 percent or less of the calories from fat.

When you find the grams of Sugars in a product, be sure to compare it to the grams of Total Carbohydrate. For example, if a cup of cereal has 32g Total Carbohydrate and 16g of Sugars, that means 50 percent of the carbohydrate in the cereal comes from sugar. Try to choose foods with 25 percent or less grams of sugars, so that you make food choices with lower amounts of sugars. Use this guideline only for food items where sugar is added to the foods. Items such as milk, yogurt, or fruit have naturally occurring sugar and do not fall into this category unless sugar has been added to the product.

Fiber grams are also part of Total Carbohydrate. Choose higher fiber foods by selecting those that contain 4 or more grams of fiber per serving.

The Glycemic Index

The glycemic index (GI) measures how a food with carbohydrate raises blood glucose. Foods are ranked on a scale from 0–100, based on a comparison to a reference food. Using the GI involves choosing foods that have a low or medium GI more often, and limiting foods known to have a high GI. Examples of carbohydrate foods with a low GI include dried beans and legumes, nonstarchy vegetables, most whole fruits, and many whole-grain breads and cereals. Foods that do not contain carbohydrates (such as meats and fats) do not have a GI. Foods that are good sources of fiber tend to have a lower GI. In general, the less processed a food is, the lower the GI. The GI of a food can be affected by its degree of ripeness, the amount and type of processing a food has sustained, or the method in which a food has been cooked. For example, a very ripe piece of fruit will have a higher GI than one that is not as ripe. Pasta that is cooked al dente has a lower GI than soft cooked pasta.

When it comes to meal planning for pre-diabetes or diabetes, there is no right way that works for everyone. The American Diabetes Association recommends using methods such as carbohydrate counting or food exchanges as the key means for monitoring total carbohydrate intake. The use of low GI as a secondary method may provide a modest additional benefit for glycemic control. If you choose to use the GI as a meal-planning tool, keep in mind the total amount of carbohydrate that you eat is still the most important factor. For more information about the glycemic index go to: *www.joslin.org* or *www.mendosa.com/gilists.htm.*

Grocery Lists and Your Kitchen Makeover

Having a plan and the right foods on hand is the best way to keep you eating healthier. If you don't have a good plan and leave things up to chance, you could make poor food choices. Grabbing fast food or take-out meals at the last minute usually means you will be eating fewer vegetables, fresh fruit, or whole-grain foods. At the same time, you will be consuming plenty of calories, fat, and refined or highly processed foods.

Set aside some time each week to plan your meals. If you work or have a very busy schedule, a good time to plan or shop may be your day off or a quiet time of the day. A little bit of time invested in meal planning saves overall time and money throughout the week.

Keep a weekly shopping list visible and handy; when you think of food items you need, write them on your list. Each time you plan, consider what meals and snacks you will need for the coming week. As you develop a shopping list, take stock of the types of foods you have in your kitchen cabinets, refrigerator, and freezer, then decide what type of items need to be added to your grocery list.

Having plenty of healthy food choices available all of the time helps you avoid the pitfalls of eating too many empty-calorie foods that get in the way of weight loss or managing your pre-diabetes.

TWENTY FOODS TO ALWAYS HAVE ON HAND

1. Vegetables: Any fresh, frozen, or reduced-sodium canned
2. Fruits: Any fresh, frozen (unsweetened), or canned (juice- or water-packed)
3. Whole-grain bread
4. High-fiber (low-sugar) cereals with 4g or more fiber per serving
5. Canned beans, dry beans, or lentils: Any variety
6. Boneless, skinless chicken or turkey breast
7. Egg substitutes or egg whites
8. Tuna or salmon canned in water
9. Low-fat cheese or cheese sticks—choose 1–1½ percent–fat varieties
10. Nonstick cooking spray
11. Dried herbs and spices: Any single varieties or mixes made without the addition of salt
12. Dry-roasted or raw nuts: walnuts and almonds are good choices
13. Noncaloric sweetener

14. Reduced-fat mayonnaise or salad dressing
15. Low-sodium chicken, vegetable, or beef broth
16. Leafy lettuce varieties or bagged salad mixes using leafy varieties
17. One or more whole grains: quinoa, amaranth, barley, bulgur, kasha, brown rice, or whole-grain pasta
18. Canned tomatoes or stewed canned tomatoes
19. Fat-free yogurt: plain, vanilla, or fruit-flavored, artificially sweetened
20. Whole-grain crackers

When you go shopping, let your shopping list guide you and stick to your list as much as possible. The healthiest foods are found around the perimeter of the store, and everything else is found in the aisles. Spend most of your time shopping around the perimeter.

Make Over Your Food Supply

Making over your kitchen food supply does not have to be extreme, costly, or stressful. You can gradually make over your kitchen cupboards by phasing out foods of lesser nutritional quality with newer ones that have more health benefits or lower calories. As you run out of items that you already have, replace the item with something new.

▼ **SUGGESTIONS FOR SWITCHING TO HEALTHIER FOODS**

Instead of:	Replace it with:
Garlic or Onion Salt	Fresh Garlic or Onion
Fruit Juices	Fresh Fruit
All-Purpose Flour	Whole-Wheat or Rye Flour
Vegetable Oil	Olive or Canola Oil
Sour Cream	Plain Low-Fat Yogurt
Buttery Snack Crackers	Whole-Grain Crackers
Cookies	Graham Crackers
Potato Chips	Popcorn (make your own)
Half Gallon of Ice Cream	Single-Serving, Reduced-Calorie Ice Cream
Bacon	Thin-Sliced, Low-Fat Ham

Helping Your Children Eat Healthier

Parents play a key role in teaching their children how to make healthier food choices. Learning healthy eating habits starts at home. You can help by creating a healthy home environment that offers nutritious options for meals and snacks. Show your child, through example, that eating right does not mean giving up good food. If you have a picky eater or your child is not on board with your healthy eating efforts, here are a few tips that may help:

- Include your child in the entire process by letting him choose healthy foods or snacks at the grocery store.
- Let your child help out in the kitchen with the preparation of a nutritious meal or snack. Children generally like to eat foods that they had a hand in making themselves.
- Keep junk foods out of the house. Your child won't be able to eat unhealthy snacks if you don't buy them.
- Look for ways to add nutritious ingredients into foods your child already likes to eat. For example, add fresh fruit to pancakes or finely chopped vegetables into spaghetti sauce.
- Keep healthy snacks visible and on hand for after-school snacks.
- Learn how to make healthy foods or snacks look more attractive by cutting up food into different shapes, adding bright colors, or creating fun faces out of fruit and vegetables. Nourish Interactive is a website with fun and kid-friendly tips to encourage healthy eating: *www .nourishinteractive.com/blog*.

Food as a Motivator

Have you ever offered food as a way to comfort, reward, or punish your child? Many parents have done this at one time or another, even if their intentions were good at the time. In some families, when the child does something worthy of praise, they are rewarded with a special dessert or ice cream. Conversely, when they have misbehaved, the dessert or special treat is withheld.

Using food as punishment or reward sends a powerful message to a child, even a very young one! Now is the time to find another way to reward or praise your child. There are plenty of ways to provide comfort or praise without the use of food. A reward system can be a motivator for making positive changes or keeping your child on track. If you decide to incorporate a reward system, start thinking of ways to provide small rewards that do not include food in the process. To provide praise for a job well done, perhaps a special outing, more time spent with you, or a chance to "earn" a special item may keep the momentum going.

Remember, although having better eating habits is a key component in the management of childhood pre-diabetes, perfection is not essential! Like adults, children have eating habits that will take time to change for the better, so be understanding, supportive, and patient. Celebrate and praise your child for the things that are working well. A positive attitude will make your child become a willing partner in the task of caring for his pre-diabetes!

Tips for Dining Out

For many Americans, work schedules and busy lifestyles have made dining out a common and frequent occurrence. Eating out can present lots of challenges when your goals are to maintain a healthy eating plan and lose weight. As with other aspects of managing your health, it's important to plan and learn about strategies for healthier eating when you go out to eat. Many people consider restaurant meals a special occasion and this can mean a time to splurge on desserts or rich foods. If you dine out frequently, viewing meals out as special occasions will sabotage your efforts to eat healthier. Take a closer look at how often you dine out, the type of food you order, and how much food you eat. Some of the pitfalls with eating out include frequent visits to fast-food restaurants or simply eating out often because you do not keep enough healthy foods available at home.

Avoiding Hidden Fats

It's no secret that many restaurant foods include plenty of oils, butter, cream, sauces, or cheeses in their preparation. Fats contribute to the flavor and taste of food, but that's where lots of extra calories come in. Foods prepared with large amounts of fat will have a higher caloric content. Healthy salad greens, for example, can end up being very high in calories if laden with large amounts of salad dressing and toppings.

The Portion Problem

One of the biggest challenges with eating out is coping with the large portions served. Unfortunately getting more food is considered a greater value, as evidenced by value meals, all-you-can-eat, or dollar incentives for extra-large options. When you eat out, be prepared to receive large portions, and have a strategy of your own to deal with this situation. If you know too much food is served at a particular restaurant, try ordering from the appetizer, soup, or salad section of the menu. Ask for a container when your meal is served and put ⅓ to ½ of the meal in the container before you start eating. You'll eat much less food that way, and have an extra meal to take home and eat later.

The best restaurant menu picks include:

- Dishes prepared with tomato sauces rather than cream sauces
- Grilled, poached, or broiled fish or poultry dishes
- Grilled or broiled meats served without gravies or sauces
- Vegetables that have been steamed or lightly sautéed
- Broth-based soups instead of cream soups
- Salads with dressing on the side and minus the extras such as cheese and croutons

ALERT

Restaurant meals can sound healthy, but be on the lookout for extra fats that may be added to the food. Cream sauces, melted cheese, sour cream, or stir-frying can add extra calories. A mere teaspoon of oil or butter provides 45–50 calories. You can take some of the guess-work out of choosing from a menu when you ask how a dish is prepared. Having this information can help you decide whether it fits into your healthy eating plan.

What about Alcohol?

When it comes to alcohol and your health, the optimal word is always moderation. Consider the facts about alcohol and decide whether including alcohol on a moderate basis fits into your pre-diabetes management plan.

Alcohol does not provide any essential nutrients, but it is a source of calories. If you drink and are having difficulty losing weight, do not overlook the calories that alcohol adds to your overall intake. Alcohol can impact blood lipid levels and elevate triglycerides. Both of these health issues may already be a source of concern for you.

It is perfectly okay to add a small amount of alcohol in certain recipes. A bit of wine or flavored liqueur can enhance the flavor of the food, and can be incorporated as a low-fat cooking ingredient or marinade. When cooked, the alcohol content diminishes, but the flavor remains.

QUESTION

What does alcohol "in moderation" mean?
Moderation is considered to be two drinks a day for men and one drink a day for women. One drink is a 12-ounce beer, 5-ounce glass of wine, or 1½ ounces of distilled spirits. Beverages with mixers (sodas, juices, etc.) have more carbohydrates. If you use mixers, lower the calories and carbohydrates by using club soda, mineral water, diet soda, or diet tonic water in the drink.

Making Recipe Adjustments for Your New Cooking Style

Your favorite recipes can be adjusted to lower fat, salt, or sugar content, yet still maintain good taste. Recipes that are cooked on the stovetop rather than baked can often turn out quite well with a simple reduction in sugar, salt, or fat. It is possible to substitute low-fat or low-sodium ingredients in certain recipes. As an example, using 1% milk instead of whole milk in a pudding recipe lowers fat and calories without significantly altering the taste.

Some of the recipes found in this cookbook may contain ingredients such as butter or salt in small amounts. These ingredients are usually part of a recipe because they improve the flavor of a food or aid in the baking process. When baking bread, cookies, or cakes, salt is usually required in the leavening process and should not be eliminated. If you must eliminate all butter from your diet, most recipes can use soft spread margarines or vegetable oil as a substitute. You and your dietitian can decide whether it is appropriate to include these ingredients in small quantities or make a substitution.

The recipes for baked desserts found in this cookbook have different methods for addressing sugar. Some recipes will simply have a reduction in the total amount of sugar used. There are other recipes that use a different type of sugar that has caloric value, such as honey or maple syrup. When these are used in the place of sugar, a lesser quantity is used; therefore, the end product is lower in sugar, but not sugar-free. Lastly, some recipes have a combination of an artificial sweetener with a very small amount of regular sugar. As you work with these or with your own recipes, you will learn how to adjust ingredients to get good results.

QUESTION

Can sugar be eliminated from my favorite cake and cookie recipes?
Completely eliminating sugar from baked desserts can be tricky. Although sugar is an empty-calorie food, it does serve as an important ingredient in certain baked foods by enhancing the flavor, texture, and appearance of the end product. When sugar is reduced or replaced with an artificial sweetener in a cake or cookie recipe, the result can be very different and not what you were hoping for. The baked good can be denser, lack a golden brown color, or have a flavor unlike the original recipe.

Tips for Replacing or Reducing Sugar and Fat

Try reducing a standard recipe's sugar content by 25–50 percent. It's usually best to start with a smaller reduction (25 percent) and gradually decrease the amount of sugar each time the product is made. Be sure to note whether the properties of the food have any significant or undesirable changes, then adjust as needed.

Use puréed, unsweetened fruit or fruit juices to replace some or all of the sugar in a recipe.

Honey or maple syrup are sugars and will affect blood sugar; however, either can add sweetness to a food. Carbohydrates and calories can be reduced in a recipe if you use a smaller amount of these sugars in a recipe.

Many recipes can withstand up to a 50 percent reduction in fat. To replace fat, but not volume, try using plain yogurt, applesauce, mashed ripe banana, or other puréed fruit for half of the oil or shortening called for in a recipe. If the product requires sweetness in addition to volume, applesauce or mashed ripe banana make good options.

Using Sugar Substitutes

Sugar substitutes are never mandatory when you have pre-diabetes, but they can offer options to those who wish to use them. Using a sugar substitute in a recipe can slash sugar content and a significant amount of calories. When using sugar substitutes in baking, keep in mind that sweetness is being added to the food, but other traits unique to a baked product (volume, texture, golden-brown color) may be altered.

The sweeteners listed below are all approved by the FDA. They vary in taste, uses, and suitability for cooking or baking. You will need to do a taste test on your own to decide which ones are best for you.

▼ **SUGAR SUBSTITUTES**

Sweetener	Brand Name	Notes
Saccharin	Sweet'N Low® or Sugar Twin®	Saccharin can leave a bitter aftertaste, and may need to be combined with other sweeteners to improve taste when used in cooking. 24 packets replaces 1 cup of sugar.
Aspartame	Equal® or NutraSweet®	High temperatures diminish sweetness, making this product less suitable for baking. Aspartame contains phenylalanine, which can be harmful to people with the rare disease phenylketonuria (PKU), and it must be avoided by them.
Sucralose	Splenda®	There are several baking products using sucralose, including a granular version that measures cup for cup with sugar. There are also half sugar and brown sugar blends, which contain sugar, so adjust accordingly.
Stevia	Truvia®, PureVia®	Look for brands of stevia that use a purified portion of the stevia leaf known as rebaudioside A. Sugar to stevia ratios vary with each brand, so follow recommendations by the manufacturer if using in cooking or baking.

Cooking Styles

There are many ways to prepare foods that not only preserve nutrients and good taste but also minimize the use of sugar, salt, and fat. A little creativity with spices, herbs, or combining foods together in unconventional ways makes food more flavorful without the addition of extra fat, sodium, or calories. Stir-frying, broiling, and slow cooking are examples of techniques that are time saving and result in more healthful food.

Stir-frying uses a very small amount of oil and cooks foods quickly at a high heat. It allows you to combine several foods together for a quick and healthy meal. Foods that work well using the stir-fry method include vegetables, poultry, meats, fish, and cooked grains. When stir-frying, choose oil with a high smoke point such as canola or peanut oil to allow for a high cooking temperature. Remember to use as little oil as possible; usually 1–2 teaspoons will do. Stir-fried foods from a restaurant menu may be very different from a home-prepared version. Before selecting a restaurant stir-fried dish, ask how the food is prepared and how much oil is being used.

Broiling or grilling involves cooking foods on a rack to allow fats to drip to a pan or flame below. Most meats, poultry, or fish can be grilled or broiled. Broiling instead of cooking in oil can reduce fat and calories. When using an outdoor grill, use aluminum foil to minimize the direct contact of food with the flame, and be sure to prevent foods from charring or overbrowning.

Slow cookers are often overlooked, but can be very helpful in the preparation of healthy meals. They are extremely easy to use and can save a lot of time in the kitchen. Foods are placed in the slow cooker early in the day and allowed to cook at a low temperature for several hours or more. Meals made in a slow cooker do not require the addition of fats, and the slow cooking helps tenderize tougher cuts of meat. Soups, sauces, and stews are just a few examples of the items you can cook in a slow cooker.

CHAPTER 7

Breakfast Fare

Egg White Pancakes

NUTRITIONAL ANALYSIS (per serving)

Calories: **197**   Protein: **13g**   Carbohydrates: **31g**   Fat: **3g**   Saturated Fat: **1g**   Cholesterol: **0mg**   Sodium: **120mg**
Fiber: **4g**   PCF Ratio: **27-61-12**   Exchange Approx.: **1 Free Sweet, 1 Lean**

INGREDIENTS | **SERVES 2**

4 egg whites

½ cup oatmeal

4 teaspoons reduced-calorie or low-sugar strawberry jam

1 teaspoon powdered sugar

Creative Toppings

Experiment with toast and pancake toppings. Try a tablespoon of raisins, almonds, apples, bananas, berries, nut butters (limit these to 1 teaspoon per serving), peanuts, pears, walnuts, or wheat germ.

1. Put all the ingredients, except powdered sugar, in blender and process until smooth.

2. Preheat a small nonstick pan treated with cooking spray over medium heat. Pour half of the mixture into pan. Cook for 4–5 minutes.

3. Flip the pancake and cook for another 4 minutes, until the inside is cooked. Repeat using remaining batter for second pancake. Dust each pancake with powdered sugar, if using.

Buckwheat Pancakes

NUTRITIONAL ANALYSIS (per serving)

Calories: 220   Protein: 11g   Carbohydrates: 44g   Fat: 1g   Saturated Fat: 0g   Cholesterol: 1mg   Sodium: 200mg
Fiber: 5g   PCF Ratio: 76-19-5   Exchange Approx.: 2 Starches, ½ Skim Milk, ½ Fruit

INGREDIENTS | SERVES 2

1 cup whole-wheat flour
½ cup buckwheat flour
1½ teaspoons baking powder
2 egg whites
¼ cup apple juice concentrate
1¼–1½ cups skim milk

1. Sift the flours and baking powder together.

2. In a medium bowl, combine the egg whites, apple juice concentrate, and 1¼ cups milk.

3. Add the milk mixture to dry ingredients and mix well, but do not overmix. Add remaining milk if necessary to reach desired consistency.

4. Cook pancakes in nonstick skillet or on griddle treated with nonstick spray over medium heat, about 1–2 minutes each side.

Berry Puff Pancakes

NUTRITIONAL ANALYSIS (per serving)

Calories: 186   Protein: 5g   Carbohydrates: 37g   Fat: 2g   Saturated Fat: 1g   Cholesterol: 71mg   Sodium: 89mg
Fiber: 3g   PCF Ratio: 65-18-17   Exchange Approx.: 1 Starch, ½ Fruit

INGREDIENTS | SERVES 6

2 large whole eggs

1 large egg white

½ cup skim milk

½ cup all-purpose flour

1 tablespoon granulated sugar

⅛ teaspoon sea salt

2 cups fresh berries such as raspberries, blackberries, boysenberries, blueberries, strawberries, or a combination

1 tablespoon powdered sugar

Syrup Substitutes

Spreading 2 teaspoons of your favorite Smucker's Low-Sugar jam or jelly on a waffle or pancake not only gives you a sweet topping, it can be one of your Free Exchange List choices for the day.

1. Preheat the oven to 450°F. Treat a 10" ovenproof skillet or deep pie pan with nonstick spray. Once oven is heated, place pan in oven for a few minutes to get hot.

2. Add the eggs and egg white to medium bowl and beat until mixed. Whisk in milk. Slowly whisk in the flour, sugar, and salt.

3. Remove preheated pan from oven and pour the batter into it. Bake for 15 minutes, then reduce the heat to 350°F and bake for an additional 10 minutes, or until batter is puffed and brown. Remove from oven and slide onto serving plate.

4. Cover with fruit and sift powdered sugar over top. Cut into 6 equal wedges and serve.

Buttermilk Pancakes

NUTRITIONAL ANALYSIS (per serving)

Calories: **143**   Protein: **6g**   Carbohydrates: **26g**   Fat: **2g**   Saturated Fat: **1g**   Cholesterol: **49mg**   Sodium: **111mg**
Fiber: **1g**   PCF Ratio: **16-74-10**   Exchange Approx.: **1½ Starches**

INGREDIENTS | SERVES 2

1 cup all-purpose flour
2 tablespoons nonfat buttermilk powder
¼ teaspoon baking soda
½ teaspoon low-salt baking powder
1 cup water

Nut Butter Batter

For a change of pace, try adding 1 Exchange amount per serving of nut butter to pancake batter and use jelly or jam instead of syrup.

1. In a large bowl, blend together all the ingredients, adding more water if necessary to get batter consistency desired.

2. Pour ¼ of batter into a medium nonstick skillet or a skillet treated with nonstick cooking spray. Cook over medium heat until bubbles appear on top half of pancake. Flip and continue cooking until center of pancake is done, about 1–2 minutes each side. Repeat process with remaining batter.

Sweet Potato Pancakes

NUTRITIONAL ANALYSIS (per serving)

Calories: **168**   Protein: **6g**   Carbohydrates: **25.87g**   Fat: **7g**   Saturated Fat: **1g**   Cholesterol: **0mg**   Sodium: **139mg**
Fiber: **3g**   PCF Ratio: **13-49-37**   Exchange Approx.: **1 Starch, 1½ Fats**

INGREDIENTS | SERVES 4

2 medium sweet potatoes
¼ cup onions, grated
1 egg
3 tablespoons whole-wheat pastry flour
½ teaspoon cinnamon
½ teaspoon baking powder
½ cup egg whites
2 tablespoons canola oil

1. Scrub sweet potatoes; pierce skins with fork and microwave on high for 4–5 minutes. When sweet potatoes have cooled enough to handle, scoop sweet potato out of skins; lightly mash with fork. (Should yield about 1½ cups cooked sweet potatoes.)

2. In a medium bowl, mix together the sweet potatoes, grated onion, and egg. Add in flour, cinnamon, and baking powder.

3. In separate small bowl, beat the egg whites until rounded peaks are formed. Gently fold egg whites into potato mixture.

4. Heat the oil in a medium skillet (preferably nonstick) until hot. Spoon batter onto skillet to form pancakes approximately 4" in diameter. Brown on both sides, about 3–4 minutes.

5. Serve hot with some unsweetened applesauce.

Country-Style Omelet

NUTRITIONAL ANALYSIS (per serving)

Calories: **253**   Protein: **17g**   Carbohydrates: **7g**   Fat: **17g**   Saturated Fat: **5g**   Cholesterol: **493mg**   Sodium: **221mg**
Fiber: **2g**   PCF Ratio: **27-12-61**   Exchange Approx.: **1 Vegetable, 2 Medium-Fat Meats, 3 Fats**

INGREDIENTS | SERVES 2

2 teaspoons olive oil

1 cup diced zucchini

¼ cup diced red pepper

1 cup plum tomatoes, skinned and cubed

⅛ teaspoon pepper

4 eggs

1 tablespoon Parmesan cheese

1 teaspoon minced fresh basil

1. Heat the oil in a medium nonstick skillet. Add zucchini and red pepper and sauté for 5 minutes.

2. Add tomatoes and pepper and cook uncovered for another 10 minutes, allowing fluid from tomatoes to cook down.

3. In a small bowl, whisk together the eggs, Parmesan cheese, and fresh basil; pour over the vegetables in skillet.

4. Cook over low heat until browned, approximately 10 minutes on each side.

Fruit Smoothie

The Nutritional Analysis and Fruit Exchange for this recipe will depend on your choice of fruit. Otherwise, allow ½ Skim Milk Exchange and ½ Misc. Food Exchange. The wheat germ adds fiber, but at less than 20 calories a serving, it can count as 1 Free Exchange.

Put all the ingredients into blender or food processor and process until thick and smooth.

INGREDIENTS | SERVES 1

1 cup skim milk

2 Exchange servings of any diced fruit

1 tablespoon honey

4 teaspoons toasted wheat germ

6 large ice cubes

Batch 'Em

Make large batches of smoothies so you can keep single servings in the freezer. Get out a serving as you begin to get ready for your day. This should give the smoothie time to thaw enough for you to stir it when you're ready to have breakfast.

Yogurt Fruit Smoothie

NUTRITIONAL ANALYSIS (per serving)

Calories: 149   Protein: 10g   Carbohydrates: 26g   Fat: 1g   Saturated Fat: 0g   Cholesterol: 2mg   Sodium: 96mg
Fiber: 2g   PCF Ratio: 25-67-8   Exchange Approx.: 1 Milk, 1 Fruit

INGREDIENTS | SERVES 2

1 cup plain low-fat yogurt
½ cup sliced strawberries
½ cup orange juice
½ cup nectarines, peeled and sliced
2 tablespoons ground flax seed

Put all the ingredients in blender and process until smooth.

Variations and Combos

You can vary this smoothie by substituting other fruits of your choice. Good combinations are strawberry and banana, strawberry and kiwi, or banana and peach. Keep portions of each fruit to no more than ½ cup.

Tofu Smoothie

NUTRITIONAL ANALYSIS (per serving)

Calories: 319   Protein: 20g   Carbohydrates: 35g   Fat: 11g   Saturated Fat: 2g   Cholesterol: 0mg   Sodium: 19mg
Fiber: 8g   PCF Ratio: 25-44-31   Exchange Approx.: 1 Meat Substitute, 2 Fruits

INGREDIENTS | SERVES 1

1⅓ cups frozen unsweetened strawberries
½ banana
½ cup (4 ounces) silken tofu

In a food processor or blender, process all the ingredients until smooth. Add a little chilled water for thinner smoothies if desired.

Overnight Oatmeal

NUTRITIONAL ANALYSIS (per serving)

Calories: 221   Protein: 9g   Carbohydrates: 42g   Fat: 3g   Saturated Fat: 1g   Cholesterol: 1mg   Sodium: 25mg
Fiber: 6g   PCF Ratio: 15-73-11   Exchange Approx.: 1 Fruit, 1 Starch, ½ Skim Milk

INGREDIENTS | SERVES 4

1 cup steel-cut oats
14 dried apricot halves
1 dried fig
2 tablespoons golden raisins
4 cups water
½ cup Mock Cream (see Chapter 16)

1. Add all the ingredients to a slow cooker with a ceramic interior.

2. Set to low heat. Cover and cook overnight (8–9 hours).

Another Method for Cooking Oatmeal

For another way to cook steel-cut oats, place 1 cup steel-cut oats, 4 cups water, and dried fruit in medium saucepan; bring to a quick boil. Turn off the heat and cover saucepan. When cooled, place in covered container and refrigerate overnight. In the morning, the oatmeal will have absorbed all of the water. Scoop 1 portion of the oatmeal into a bowl; microwave on high for 1½–2 minutes. Add milk and serve. Heat up refrigerated leftover portions as needed; use within 3 days.

Egg Clouds on Toast

NUTRITIONAL ANALYSIS (per serving)

Calories: **57**   Protein: **4g**   Carbohydrates: **9g**   Fat: **1g**   Saturated Fat: **0g**   Cholesterol: **0mg**   Sodium: **101mg**   Fiber: **0g**   PCF Ratio: **30-63-7**   Exchange Approx.: **½ Very-Lean Fat Meat, ½ Starch**

INGREDIENTS | SERVES 1

2 egg whites

½ teaspoon sugar

1 cup water

1 tablespoon frozen apple juice concentrate

1 slice reduced-calorie oat-bran bread, lightly toasted

Tip

Additional serving suggestions: Spread 1 teaspoon of low-sugar or all-fruit spread on toast (½ Fruit Exchange) before ladling on the "clouds." For cinnamon French-style toast, sprinkle ¼ teaspoon cinnamon and ½ teaspoon powdered sugar (less than 10 calories) over top of the clouds.

1. In a copper bowl, beat the egg whites until thickened. Add sugar and continue to beat until stiff peaks form.

2. In a small saucepan, heat water and apple juice over medium heat until it just begins to boil. Reduce heat and allow mixture to simmer.

3. Drop egg whites by teaspoonful into the simmering water. Simmer for 3 minutes; turn over and simmer for an additional 3 minutes.

4. Ladle "clouds" over bread and serve immediately.

Quinoa Berry Breakfast

NUTRITIONAL ANALYSIS (per serving)

Calories: **228**   Protein: **7g**   Carbohydrates: **41g**   Fat: **5g**   Saturated Fat: **0g**   Cholesterol: **0mg**   Sodium: **2mg**
Fiber: **5g**   PCF Ratio: **12-69-19**   Exchange Approx.: **2 Starches, 1 Fruit, 1 Very-Lean Meat, 1 Fat**

INGREDIENTS	SERVES 4

1 cup quinoa
2 cups water
¼ cup walnuts
1 teaspoon cinnamon
2 cups berries

Single Serving Quick Tip

Use this basic recipe to make 4 servings at once. Refrigerate any leftover portions; microwave for 1–1½ minutes on high for single portions as needed. Use cooked quinoa within 3 days. Try other berries, nuts, or spices such as ginger or nutmeg to vary this nutritious breakfast cereal.

1. Rinse the quinoa in fine-mesh sieve before cooking. Place the quinoa, water, walnuts, and cinnamon in a 1½-quart saucepan and bring to a boil.

2. Reduce the heat to low; cover and cook for 15 minutes, or until all water has been absorbed.

3. Add the berries and serve with milk, soy milk, or sweetener if desired.

CHAPTER 8

Soups

Lentil Soup with Herbs and Lemon

NUTRITIONAL ANALYSIS (per serving)

Calories: **214** Protein: **15g** Carbohydrates: **34g** Fat: **3g** Saturated Fat: **1g** Cholesterol: **0mg** Sodium: **353mg**
Fiber: **16g** PCF Ratio: **27-61-12** Exchange Approx.: **1 Lean Meat, 2 Starches, 1 Vegetable**

INGREDIENTS | SERVES 4

1 cup lentils, soaked overnight in 1 cup water

6 cups low-fat, reduced-sodium chicken broth

1 carrot, sliced

1 stalk celery, sliced

1 yellow onion, thinly sliced

2 teaspoons olive oil

1 tablespoon dried tarragon

½ teaspoon dried oregano

Sea salt and black pepper, to taste (optional)

1 tablespoon lemon juice

4 thin slices of lemon

Believe It or Not!

Put a fork at the bottom of the pan when you cook a pot of beans. The beans will cook in half the time.

1. Drain and rinse the lentils. Add lentils and broth to a pot over medium heat; bring to a boil. Reduce heat and simmer until tender, approximately 15 minutes. (If you did not presoak the lentils, increase cooking time by about 15 minutes.)

2. While the lentils are cooking, sauté the carrot, celery, and onion in oil for 8 minutes, or until onion is golden brown. Remove from heat and set aside.

3. When lentils are tender, add the vegetables, tarragon, oregano, and salt and pepper (if using) to the pot and cook for 2 minutes.

4. Stir in lemon juice. Ladle into 4 serving bowls; garnish with lemon slices.

Tomato-Vegetable Soup

NUTRITIONAL ANALYSIS (per serving)

Calories: **158** Protein: **5g** Carbohydrates: **31g** Fat: **3g** Saturated Fat: **1g** Cholesterol: **0mg** Sodium: **349mg**

Fiber: **5g** PCF Ratio: **12-72-16** Exchange Approx.: **1½ Starches, 1 Vegetable**

INGREDIENTS | SERVES 6

1 tablespoon olive oil

2 teaspoons minced garlic

⅔ teaspoon cumin

2 carrots, chopped

2 stalks celery, diced

1 medium onion, chopped

⅔ cup unsalted tomato paste

½ teaspoon red pepper flakes

2 cups canned unsalted peeled tomatoes, with juice

⅔ teaspoon chopped fresh oregano

3 cups low-fat, reduced-sodium chicken broth

3 cups fat-free beef broth

2 cups diced potatoes

2 cups shredded cabbage

½ cup green beans

½ cup fresh or frozen corn kernels

½ teaspoon freshly cracked black pepper

¼ cup lime juice or balsamic vinegar

1. Heat the olive oil in large stockpot. Add the garlic, cumin, carrot, and celery and sauté for 1 minute. Add onion; cook until transparent, about 3–4 minutes.

2. Stir in the tomato paste and sauté until it begins to brown.

3. Add the remaining ingredients, except for the lime juice or vinegar. Bring to a boil. Reduce heat and simmer for 20–30 minutes, adding additional broth or water if needed.

4. Just before serving, add lime juice or balsamic vinegar.

Easy Measures

Consider freezing broth in an ice cube tray. Most ice cube tray sections hold ⅛ cup (2 tablespoons) of liquid. Once broth is frozen, you can transfer cubes to a freezer bag or container. This makes it easy to measure out the amount you need for recipes.

Minestrone Soup Genoese Style

NUTRITIONAL ANALYSIS (per serving)

Calories: **201** Protein: **9g** Carbohydrates: **29g** Fat: **6g** Saturated Fat: **2g** Cholesterol: **5mg** Sodium: **271mg**
Fiber: **6g** PCF Ratio: **17-56-27** Exchange Approx.: **1½ Starches, 1 Vegetable, 1 Fat**

INGREDIENTS | SERVES 6

4 cloves garlic, minced
2 tablespoons chopped basil
¼ teaspoon salt
2 tablespoons olive oil
1 ounce Romano cheese
2 cups shredded cabbage
1 cup diced zucchini
1 cup green beans, cut into 1" pieces
1 cup peeled and chopped potatoes
2 cups cooked navy beans
½ cup chopped celery
¼ cup peas, fresh or frozen
1 tablespoon tomato paste
3 cups water
Salt and pepper, to taste

1. In a medium bowl, combine the garlic, basil, and salt. Add olive oil and Romano cheese; mix well into a paste and set aside. (Using a mortar and pestle works very well.)

2. In a 4–6-quart soup pot, combine the cabbage, zucchini, green beans, potatoes, cooked navy beans, celery, peas, tomato paste, and water.

3. Bring to a boil. Reduce heat and simmer for 45–60 minutes, or until tender.

4. Mix garlic paste into soup; simmer for an additional 5 minutes. Add salt and pepper to taste and serve.

Tip

Make extra garlic paste (using first 5 ingredients and step 1) and keep refrigerated. You'll have instant garlic-cheese flavor on hand for soups, sauces, garlic bread, and pasta dishes. Garlic paste keeps in the refrigerator for up to 2 weeks.

Broccoli and Whole-Grain Pasta Soup

NUTRITIONAL ANALYSIS (per serving)

Calories: 86   Protein: 6g   Carbohydrates: 10g   Fat: 3g   Saturated Fat: 1g   Cholesterol: 9mg   Sodium: 185mg
Fiber: 2g   PCF Ratio: 25-43-32   Exchange Approx.: ½ Starch, 1 Vegetable, 1 Fat

INGREDIENTS | SERVES 6

1–3 slices bacon, cut into 1" pieces

1 tablespoon chopped onion

2 cloves garlic, minced

1 tablespoon tomato paste

3 cups water

1 cup peeled and cubed eggplant

¾ teaspoon salt

¼ teaspoon pepper

½ teaspoon oregano

8 ounces broccoli florets

1 cup whole-grain pasta shells, cooked al dente

1 ounce grated Romano cheese

1. Place the bacon, onion, and garlic in a 4-quart soup pot and brown for 5–7 minutes. Add the tomato paste, water, eggplant, salt, pepper, and oregano. Bring to a boil. Reduce heat and simmer for 20 minutes, or until the eggplant is soft cooked.

2. Add the broccoli florets and simmer for 5 minutes, until the broccoli is tender but still slightly crisp. Add cooked pasta.

3. Serve soup immediately with a sprinkling of grated cheese.

Cold Roasted Red Pepper Soup

NUTRITIONAL ANALYSIS (per serving, without salt)

Calories: **73** Protein: **5g** Carbohydrates: **9g** Fat: **4g** Saturated Fat: **1g** Cholesterol: **3mg** Sodium: **404mg**
Fiber: **3g** PCF Ratio: **21-39-40** Exchange Approx.: **½ Fat, ½ Starch**

INGREDIENTS | SERVES 4

1 teaspoon olive oil

½ cup chopped onion

3 roasted red bell peppers, seeded and chopped (see directions for Roasted Red Pepper and Plum Sauce recipe in Chapter 16)

3¼ cups low-fat, reduced-sodium chicken broth

½ cup nonfat plain yogurt

½ teaspoon sea salt (optional)

4 sprigs fresh basil (optional)

1. Heat a saucepan over medium-high heat. Add the olive oil and onion and sauté for 3–4 minutes until transparent.

2. Add the peppers and broth. Bring to a boil. Reduce heat and simmer for 15 minutes. Remove from heat; purée in blender or food processor until smooth. Allow to cool.

3. Stir in the yogurt and salt if using and chill well in refrigerator. Garnish the soup with fresh basil sprigs, if desired.

Nutty Greek Snapper Soup

NUTRITIONAL ANALYSIS (per serving)

Calories: **309**   Protein: **39g**   Carbohydrates: **25g**   Fat: **6g**   Saturated Fat: **1g**   Cholesterol: **46mg**   Sodium: **240mg**
Fiber: **2g**   PCF Ratio: **50-33-17**   Exchange Approx.: **4 Lean Meats, 1 Skim Milk, 1 Vegetable**

INGREDIENTS | **SERVES 4**

1 pound (16 ounces) red snapper fillet

2 large cucumbers

4 green onions, chopped

4 cups nonfat plain yogurt

1 cup packed fresh parsley, basil, cilantro, arugula, and chives, mixed

3 tablespoons lime juice

Salt and pepper, to taste (optional)

¼ cup chopped walnuts

Herb sprigs for garnish (optional)

Tip

You can make this soup using leftover fish or substitute halibut, cod, or sea bass for the snapper.

1. Rinse red snapper fillet and pat dry with paper towels. Broil the fillet until opaque through the thickest part, about 4 minutes on each side depending on the thickness of fillet. Let cool. (Alternatives would be to steam or poach the fillet.)

2. Peel and halve cucumbers and scoop out and discard seeds. Cut into 1" pieces.

3. Put half of the cucumber with green onions in the bowl of a food processor and pulse to coarsely chop. Transfer to a large bowl.

4. Add the remaining cucumber, yogurt, and herb leaves to the food processor and process until smooth and frothy. (Alternatively, you can grate cucumbers, finely mince green onion and herbs, and stir together with yogurt in large bowl.)

5. Stir in the lime juice and season with salt and pepper to taste, if using. Cover and refrigerate for at least 1 hour or up to 8 hours; the longer the soup cools, the more the flavors will mellow.

6. While the soup cools, break the cooled red snapper fillet into large chunks, discarding any skin or bones.

7. Ladle chilled soup into shallow bowls and add red snapper. Sprinkle chopped walnuts over soup, garnish with herb sprigs, and serve.

White Bean and Escarole Soup

NUTRITIONAL ANALYSIS (per serving)

Calories: 163   Protein: 11g   Carbohydrates: 27g   Fat: 2g   Saturated Fat: 0g   Cholesterol: 7mg   Sodium: 349mg
Fiber: 9g   PCF Ratio: 26-64-10   Exchange Approx.: 1½ Starches, ½ Vegetable, 1½ Very-Lean Meats, 2 Fats

INGREDIENTS | SERVES 6

1 cup dry navy beans

3 cups water

1 cup chopped onion

½ cup peeled and chopped potato

1 clove garlic, minced

3 ounces Canadian bacon, cut in ½" cubes

2½ cups water

½ teaspoon salt

¼ teaspoon pepper

1 teaspoon vegetable oil

8 ounces escarole, coarsely chopped

1. Place the dry beans and 3 cups of water in a medium saucepan. Bring to a boil. Remove from heat. Allow beans to soak several hours or overnight.

2. Drain the beans, place them in a pressure cooker with the onion, potatoes, garlic, Canadian bacon, 2½ cups water, salt, pepper, and vegetable oil. Close cover securely, place pressure regulator on vent pipe, and cook for 30 minutes with pressure regulator rocking slowly. (If using an electric pressure cooker, follow manufacturer instructions.) Let pressure drop on its own.

3. Add the chopped escarole and simmer for 5–10 minutes, until escarole is wilted and cooked tender.

Slow-Cooker Method

This soup can also be prepared using a slow cooker. Soak beans as described in step 1 and then drain. Add beans, onion, potatoes, garlic, Canadian bacon, and 2½ cups water to a slow cooker. Cook for 8–10 hours. At end of cooking, add the escarole; simmer for 5–10 minutes, until escarole is wilted and tender. Add salt and pepper to taste.

Fresh Tomato Basil Soup

NUTRITIONAL ANALYSIS (per serving)

Calories: **87**   Protein: **3g**   Carbohydrates: **12g**   Fat: **4g**   Saturated Fat: **2g**   Cholesterol: **10mg**   Sodium: **449mg**
Fiber: **3g**   PCF Ratio: **13-50-37**   Exchange Approx.: **2 Vegetables, 1 Fat**

INGREDIENTS | SERVES 6

1 tablespoon butter
¼ cup chopped onion
4 cups (2 pounds) crushed tomatoes
¼ cup fresh basil leaves, loosely chopped
1 cup low-sodium chicken broth
2 ounces reduced-fat (Neufchâtel) cream cheese
Fresh ground pepper, to taste

1. Melt the butter in a soup pot. Add the onion and sauté for 2–3 minutes until soft.

2. Add the crushed tomatoes, basil, and chicken broth.

3. Bring to a boil. Reduce heat and cook for 15 minutes.

4. Remove from heat and stir in the cream cheese until melted.

5. Transfer to a food processor or blender and purée until smooth. Depending on size of processor or blender, you may need to purée a partial portion at a time.

Winter Squash and Red Pepper Soup

NUTRITIONAL ANALYSIS (per serving)

Calories: **137**   Protein: **3g**   Carbohydrates: **24g**   Fat: **3g**   Saturated Fat: **1g**   Cholesterol: **0mg**   Sodium: **445mg**
Fiber: **6g**   PCF Ratio: **10-70-20**   Exchange Approx.: **1 Starch, 1 Vegetable, ½ Fat**

INGREDIENTS | SERVES 6

1 large winter squash
1 tablespoon olive oil
1 cup chopped onions
1 tablespoon chopped garlic
4 ounces roasted red pepper
3 cups low-sodium chicken broth
½ cup dry white wine
2 teaspoons sugar
1 teaspoon cinnamon
½ teaspoon ginger
1 tablespoon reduced-fat sour cream (optional)

1. Wash and cut the squash in half; core out the seeds. Place face down on oiled 9" × 13" glass baking dish and bake at 400°F for 50–60 minutes, or until squash is cooked tender. When cool enough to handle, scoop squash out of shells and set aside. Yield should be about 3½ cups squash.

2. In a large nonstick skillet heat the olive oil. Add the onions and garlic and sauté until tender and continue to cook until the onions are soft and have turned brown (caramelized), about 8–10 minutes.

3. Add the roasted pepper and chicken broth and simmer for 16 minutes.

4. Add the cooked winter squash, white wine, sugar, cinnamon, and ginger and simmer for 5 minutes.

5. Transfer the mixture to a food processor or blender and purée until smooth. Depending on size of processor or blender, you may need to purée a partial portion at a time. If desired, stir in reduced-fat sour cream and serve.

Rich and Creamy Sausage-Potato Soup

NUTRITIONAL ANALYSIS (per serving)

Calories: **326**   Protein: **17g**   Carbohydrates: **53g**   Fat: **6g**   Saturated Fat: **2g**   Cholesterol: **19mg**   Sodium: **259mg**
Fiber: **3g**   PCF Ratio: **20-64-16**   Exchange Approx.:**1 Fat, ½ Medium-Fat Meat, 1 Starch, 1½ Skim Milks, 1 Vegetable**

INGREDIENTS | SERVES 2

1 teaspoon olive oil

½ teaspoon butter

½ cup chopped onion, steamed

1 clove dry-roasted garlic (see Chicken with Portobello Mushrooms and Roasted Garlic recipe in Chapter 10)

1 ounce crumbled cooked chorizo

¼ teaspoon celery seed

2 Yukon Gold potatoes, peeled and diced into 1" pieces

½ cup fat-free chicken broth

1½ cups Mock Cream (see Chapter 16)

1 teaspoon white wine vinegar

1 teaspoon vanilla extract

Fresh parsley, to taste (optional)

Sea salt and freshly ground black pepper, to taste (optional)

1. In a saucepan over medium heat, heat the olive oil and butter. Add the onion, roasted garlic, chorizo, celery seed, and potatoes; sauté until heated, about 5 minutes.

2. Add the chicken broth and bring to a boil. Cover saucepan, reduce heat, and maintain simmer for 10 minutes, or until potatoes are tender. Add mock cream and heat.

3. Remove pan from burner and stir in vinegar and vanilla. Garnish with parsley and add salt and pepper to taste.

Skim the Fat

You can remove fat from soups and stews by dropping ice cubes into the pot. The fat will cling to the cubes as you stir. Be sure to take out the cubes before they melt. Fat also clings to lettuce leaves; simply sweep them over the top of the soup. Discard ice cubes or leaves when done.

Chicken Corn Chowder

NUTRITIONAL ANALYSIS (per serving)

Calories: 193 Protein: 17g Carbohydrates: 21g Fat: 5g Saturated Fat: 3g Cholesterol: 39mg Sodium: 155mg
Fiber: 2g PCF Ratio: 22-36-42 Exchange Approx.: 1½ Very-Lean Meats, ½ Starch, 1 Vegetable, ½ Skim Milk, ½ High-Fat Meat

INGREDIENTS | SERVES 10

1 pound boneless, skinless chicken breast, cut into chunks

1 medium onion, chopped

1 red bell pepper, diced

1 large potato, diced

2 (16-ounce) cans low-fat, reduced-sodium chicken broth

1 (8¾-ounce) can unsalted cream-style corn

½ cup all-purpose flour

2 cups skim milk

4 ounces Cheddar cheese, diced

½ teaspoon sea salt

Freshly ground pepper, to taste

½ cup processed bacon bits

Tip

To trim down the fat in this recipe, use a reduced-fat cheese, such as Cabot's 50 Percent Light Cheddar.

1. Spray a large soup pot with nonstick cooking spray and heat on medium setting until hot.

2. Add the chicken, onion, and bell pepper and sauté over medium heat until chicken is browned and vegetables are tender, about 10 minutes.

3. Stir in the potatoes and broth and bring to a boil. Reduce heat and simmer, covered, for 20 minutes. Stir in corn.

4. In a medium bowl, combine the flour and milk until blended and then gradually stir into the pot. Increase heat to medium and cook until the mixture comes to a boil, then reduce heat and simmer until soup is thickened, stirring constantly, about 5 minutes.

5. Add the cheese and stir until melted and blended in. Add salt and pepper to taste and sprinkle with bacon bits before serving.

Salmon Chowder

NUTRITIONAL ANALYSIS (per serving)

Calories: 364 Protein: 20g Carbohydrates: 61g Fat: 6g Saturated Fat: 2g Cholesterol: 28mg Sodium: 199mg
Fiber: 7g PCF Ratio: 22-65-14 Exchange Approx.: ½ Fat, 2 Starches, 2 Lean Meats, 2 Vegetables, ½ Skim Milk

INGREDIENTS | SERVES 4

1 (7½-ounce) can unsalted salmon
2 teaspoons butter
1 medium onion, chopped
2 stalks celery, chopped
1 sweet green pepper, seeded and chopped
1 clove garlic, minced
4 carrots, peeled and diced
4 small potatoes, peeled and diced
1 cup fat-free chicken broth
1 cup water
½ teaspoon cracked black pepper
½ teaspoon dill seed
1 cup diced zucchini
1 cup Mock Cream (see Chapter 16)
1 (8¾-ounce) can unsalted cream-style corn
Freshly ground black pepper, to taste
½ cup chopped fresh parsley (optional)

1. Drain and flake the salmon; discard the liquid.

2. In large nonstick saucepan, melt the butter over medium heat. Add the onion, celery, green pepper, garlic, and carrots and sauté, stirring often, until tender, about 5 minutes.

3. Add the potatoes, broth, water, pepper, and dill seed. Bring to boil. Reduce heat, cover, and simmer for 20 minutes, or until potatoes are tender.

4. Add the zucchini and simmer, covered, for another 5 minutes.

5. Add salmon, mock cream, corn, and pepper and cook over low heat just until heated through, about 3 minutes. Just before serving, add parsley, if desired.

CHAPTER 9

Meat Dishes

Beef Broth: Easy Slow-Cooker Method

INGREDIENTS	YIELDS ABOUT 3 CUPS BROTH; SERVING SIZE: ½ CUP

1 pound lean round steak
1 onion, chopped
2 carrots, peeled and chopped
2 celery stalks and leaves, chopped
1 bay leaf
4 sprigs parsley
6 black peppercorns
¼ cup dry white wine
4½ cups water

Trade Secrets

Some chefs swear that a hearty beef broth requires oven-roasted bones. Place bones on a roasting tray and bake in a 425°F oven for 30–60 minutes. Blot fat from bones before adding to the rest of the broth ingredients. You may need to reduce the amount of water in your slow cooker, which will produce a more concentrated broth.

1. Cut the beef into several pieces and then add to a slow cooker with all the other ingredients. Use high setting until mixture reaches a boil, then reduce heat to low. Allow to simmer, covered, overnight, or up to 16 hours.

2. Remove beef and drain on paper towels to absorb any fat. Strain the broth, discarding any meat and vegetables. (You don't want to eat vegetables cooked directly with the beef because they will have absorbed too much of the residue fat.)

3. Put the broth in a covered container and refrigerate for several hours or overnight; this allows time for fat to congeal on top of broth. Remove hardened fat and discard. (When you remove fat from broth, the Exchange Approximation for it will be a Free Exchange.) Broth will keep in refrigerator for a few days. Freeze any broth you won't use within that time.

Stovetop Grilled Beef Loin

NUTRITIONAL ANALYSIS (per serving)

Calories: 105   Protein: 15g   Carbohydrates: 1g   Fat: 4g   Saturated Fat: 1g   Cholesterol: 2mg   Sodium: 27mg
Fiber: 0g   PCF Ratio: 58-5-37   Exchange Approx.: 2½ Lean Meats

INGREDIENTS | **YIELDS 1 (5-OUNCE) LOIN; SERVING SIZE: 2½ OUNCES**

1 lean beef tenderloin fillet, no more than 1" thick

½ teaspoon paprika

1½ teaspoons garlic powder

⅛ teaspoon cracked black pepper

¼ teaspoon onion powder

Pinch to ⅛ teaspoon cayenne pepper (according to taste)

⅛ teaspoon dried oregano

⅛ teaspoon dried thyme

½ teaspoon brown sugar

½ teaspoon olive oil

Weights and Measures: Before and After

Exchanges are based on cooking weight of meats; however, in the case of lean pork loin trimmed of all fat, very little weight is lost during the cooking process. Therefore, amounts given for raw pork loin in recipes equal cooked weights. If you find your cooking method causes more variation in weight, adjust accordingly.

1. Remove the loin from refrigerator 30 minutes before preparing it to allow it to come to room temperature. Pat meat dry with paper towels.

2. In a small bowl, mix together all dry ingredients.

3. Rub ¼ teaspoon of olive oil on each side of the fillet. (The olive oil is used in this recipe to help the "rub" adhere to the meat and to aid in the caramelization process.) Divide seasoning mixture and rub into each oiled side.

4. Heat a grill pan on high heat for 1–2 minutes, until the pan is sizzling hot. Place beef fillet in pan, reduce heat to medium-high, and cook for 3 minutes. Use tongs to turn fillet. (Be careful not to pierce meat.) Cook for another 2 minutes for medium or 3 minutes for well-done.

5. Remove from heat and let the meat rest in pan for at least 5 minutes, allowing juices to redistribute throughout meat and complete cooking process, which makes for a juicier fillet.

The Ultimate Grilled Cheeseburger Sandwich

NUTRITIONAL ANALYSIS (per serving)

Calories: 262   Protein: 17g   Carbohydrates: 15g   Fat: 15g   Saturated Fat: 5g   Cholesterol: 60mg   Sodium: 252mg
Fiber: 1.22g   PCF Ratio: 26-24-50   Exchange Approx.: 2 Lean Meats, 1 Fat, 1 Starch

INGREDIENTS | SERVES 4

1 tablespoon olive oil

1 teaspoon butter

2 thick slices of 7-Grain Bread (see Chapter 18)

1 ounce Cheddar cheese

½ pound (8 ounces) ground round

1 teaspoon Worcestershire sauce, or to taste

Fresh minced garlic, to taste

Balsamic vinegar, to taste

Toppings of your choice such as stoneground mustard, mayonnaise, etc.

The Olive Oil Factor

Once you've used an olive oil and butter mixture to butter the bread for a toasted or grilled sandwich, you'll never want to use just plain butter again! Olive oil helps make the bread crunchier and imparts a subtle taste difference to the sandwiches.

1. Preheat an indoor grill.

2. In a small bowl, combine the olive oil and butter. Use half to butter one side of each slice of bread. Place Cheddar cheese on unbuttered side of one slice of bread; top with other slice, buttered-side up.

3. In a large bowl, combine the ground round with Worcestershire sauce, garlic, and balsamic vinegar, if using. Shape mixture into 4 large, rectangular patties, a little larger than slice of bread.

4. Grill patty for 5 minutes on each side, and then cheese sandwich for 1–2 minutes per side. (If you are using a large indoor grill, position hamburger at lower end, near area where fat drains; grill cheese sandwich at higher end.)

5. Once cheese sandwich is done, separate slices of bread, being careful not to burn yourself on cheese. Top one slice with hamburger and add your choice of condiments and fixin's.

Southwest Black Bean Burgers

NUTRITIONAL ANALYSIS (per serving)

Calories: **230**   Protein: **20g**   Carbohydrates: **10g**   Fat: **12g**   Saturated Fat: **4g**   Cholesterol: **55mg**   Sodium: **15.02mg**
Fiber: **4g**   PCF Ratio: **36-18-46**   Exchange Approx.: **2½ Lean Meats, ½ Starch, 1 Fat**

INGREDIENTS | SERVES 5

1 cup cooked black beans
¼ cup chopped onion
1 teaspoon chili powder
1 teaspoon ground cumin
1 tablespoon minced fresh parsley
1 tablespoon minced fresh cilantro
½ teaspoon salt (optional)
¾ pound lean ground beef

Swapping Fresh Herbs for Dried
If you do not have fresh herbs such as parsley or cilantro available, 1 teaspoon dried can be used in place of 1 tablespoon fresh.

1. Place the beans, onion, chili powder, cumin, parsley, cilantro, and salt (if using) in a food processor. Combine ingredients using pulse setting until beans are partially puréed and all ingredients are mixed. (If using canned beans, drain and rinse first.)

2. In a separate bowl, combine the ground beef and the prepared bean mixture. Shape into 5 patties. The meat mixture is quite soft after mixing and should be chilled or partially frozen prior to cooking.

3. Grill or broil on oiled surface for about 5–7 minutes per side.

Italian Sausage

NUTRITIONAL ANALYSIS (per serving, without salt)

Calories: 135   Protein: 15g   Carbohydrates: 0g   Fat: 8g   Saturated Fat: 3g   Cholesterol: 45mg   Sodium: 27mg
Fiber: 0g   PCF Ratio: 47-0-53   Exchange Approx.: 1 Medium-Fat Meat

INGREDIENTS | **YIELDS ABOUT 2 POUNDS (32 OUNCES); SERVING SIZE: 2 OUNCES**

2 pounds (32 ounces) pork shoulder

1 teaspoon ground black pepper

1 teaspoon dried parsley

1 teaspoon Italian-style seasoning

1 teaspoon garlic powder

¾ teaspoon crushed anise seeds

⅛ teaspoon crushed red pepper flakes

½ teaspoon paprika

½ teaspoon instant minced onion flakes

1 teaspoon kosher or sea salt (optional)

1. Remove all fat from meat and cut the meat into cubes. Put in food processor and grind to desired consistency.

2. Add the remaining ingredients and mix until well blended. You can put sausage mixture in casings, but it works equally well broiled or grilled as patties.

Simple (and Smart!) Substitutions

Game meats—buffalo, venison, elk, moose—are low in fat, as are ground chicken or turkey. Substitute one of these for pork in any of the sausage recipes in this chapter.

Italian Sweet Fennel Sausage

NUTRITIONAL ANALYSIS (per serving, without salt)

Calories: **139** Protein: **15g** Carbohydrates: **1g** Fat: **8g** Saturated Fat: **3g** Cholesterol: **45mg** Sodium: **27mg**
Fiber: **0g** PCF Ratio: **46-3-51** Exchange Approx.: **1 Medium-Fat Meat**

INGREDIENTS | **YIELDS ABOUT 2 POUNDS (32 OUNCES); SERVING SIZE: 2 OUNCES**

1 tablespoon fennel seed

¼ teaspoon cayenne pepper

2 pounds (32 ounces) pork butt

½ teaspoon black pepper

2½ teaspoons crushed garlic

1 tablespoon sugar

1 teaspoon kosher or sea salt (optional)

1. Toast the fennel seeds and cayenne pepper in nonstick skillet over medium heat, stirring constantly, until seeds just begin to darken, about 2 minutes. Set aside.

2. Remove all the fat from meat and cut the meat into cubes. Put in food processor and grind to desired consistency. Add the remaining ingredients and mix until well blended. You can put sausage mixture in casings, but it works equally well broiled or grilled as patties.

Better the Second Day

Ideally, sausage is made the night before and refrigerated to allow the flavors to merge. Leftover sausage can be frozen for up to 3 months.

Mock Chorizo

NUTRITIONAL ANALYSIS (per serving, without salt)

Calories: **137**   Protein: **15g**   Carbohydrates: **1g**   Fat: **8g**   Saturated Fat: **3g**   Cholesterol: **45mg**   Sodium: **27mg**
Fiber: **0g**   PCF Ratio: **47-1-52**   Exchange Approx.: **1 Medium-Fat Meat**

INGREDIENTS | **YIELDS ABOUT 2 POUNDS (32 OUNCES); SERVING SIZE: 2 OUNCES**

2 pounds (32 ounces) lean pork
4 tablespoons chili powder
¼ teaspoon ground cloves
2 tablespoons paprika
2½ teaspoons crushed fresh garlic
1 teaspoon crushed dried oregano
3½ tablespoons cider vinegar
1 teaspoon kosher or sea salt (optional)

1. Remove all the fat from meat and cut the meat into cubes. Put in food processor and grind to desired consistency.

2. Add the remaining ingredients and mix until well blended.

3. Tradition calls for aging this sausage in an airtight container in the refrigerator for 4 days before cooking. Leftover sausage can be stored in the freezer up to 3 months.

Break from Tradition

Traditionally, chorizo is very high in fat. This chorizo recipe is a lower-fat alternative. It makes an excellent replacement for adding flavor to recipes that call for bacon. In fact, 1 or 2 ounces of chorizo can replace an entire pound of bacon in cabbage, bean, or potato soup.

Kousa (Squash Stuffed with Lamb and Rice)

NUTRITIONAL ANALYSIS (per serving)

Calories: **430** Protein: **27g** Carbohydrates: **36g** Fat: **20g** Saturated Fat: **7g** Cholesterol: **82mg** Sodium: **692mg**
Fiber: **5g** PCF Ratio: **25-33-42** Exchange Approx.: **3 Lean Meats, 1 Starch, 3 Vegetables, 3 Fats**

INGREDIENTS | SERVES 4

3 cups chopped tomatoes

1 cup chopped onion

2 cups water

½ teaspoon salt

⅛ teaspoon fresh ground pepper

2 tablespoons minced fresh mint

4 small zucchini squash (7"–8" long)

¾ pound very lean ground lamb

½ cup white rice, uncooked

2 tablespoons pine nuts

½ teaspoon salt

⅛ teaspoon allspice

⅛ teaspoon fresh ground pepper

Summer Harvest

Kousa (stuffed squash) is a traditional Lebanese dish that uses a pale green summer squash very similar to zucchini. This squash is not always easy to find, but zucchini is very abundant and works quite well. If you have a large garden crop of zucchini: Pick them small, hollow out the squash, blanch in boiling water for 2 minutes, then freeze. You'll have squash ready to stuff all year long.

1. Prepare the tomato sauce first: In a large pot, combine the tomatoes, onion, water, salt, pepper, and fresh mint. Bring to a boil. Reduce heat and simmer for 30 minutes.

2. Scrub squash and dry with paper towels. Remove stem ends of each squash and carefully core center, leaving about ¼" of shell.

3. Make the stuffing: In a medium bowl, thoroughly mix the ground lamb, rice, pine nuts, salt, allspice, and pepper.

4. Spoon stuffing into each squash, tapping bottom end of squash to get stuffing down. Fill each squash to top; stuffing should be loosely packed to allow rice to expand while cooking.

5. Place the squash in the tomato sauce, laying them on their sides. Bring sauce to a slow boil; cover and cook over low heat for 45–60 minutes, or until squash is tender and rice has cooked. Serve squash with tomato sauce spooned over top.

Baked Stuffed Kibbeh (Ground Lamb and Bulgur Wheat)

NUTRITIONAL ANALYSIS (per serving)

Calories: **226**   Protein: **18g**   Carbohydrates: **13g**   Fat: **12g**   Saturated Fat: **4g**   Cholesterol: **62mg**   Sodium: **343mg**
Fiber: **3g**   PCF Ratio: **32-22-46**   Exchange Approx.: **1 Starch, 2 Lean Meats, 2 Fats**

INGREDIENTS | SERVES 8

Cooking spray
¾ cup bulgur wheat, fine grind
2 cups boiling water
1 pound lean ground lamb
1 cup grated onion
1 teaspoon salt
¼ teaspoon pepper
Small bowl ice water
1½ tablespoons butter
¼ cup pine nuts
¼ teaspoon cinnamon
¼ teaspoon allspice
1½ tablespoons butter

Making Lean Ground Lamb

Unless you have a butcher, very lean ground lamb is difficult to find. Make it yourself using chunks of meat trimmed from a leg of lamb. Be sure to remove all visible fat from the lamb and grind twice using a medium or fine grinder blade. Removing all visible fat prevents lamb from having a strong "mutton" taste.

1. Spray 9" × 9" baking dish with cooking spray.

2. Put bulgur wheat in small bowl. Cover with boiling water and allow wheat to absorb liquid, approximately 15–20 minutes.

3. Line colander with small piece of cheesecloth. Drop bulgur wheat into cloth and drain and squeeze as much liquid out of wheat as possible.

4. Preheat oven to 350°F. On a large cutting board, combine the lamb, ½ cup grated onions, wheat, salt, and pepper and mix it with your hands, kneading together all ingredients.

5. Divide meat mixture in half. Place half in bottom of baking dish by dipping hands into ice water to spread meat mixture smoothly over bottom of dish. Cover bottom of dish completely.

6. In a small pan, melt 1½ tablespoons of butter. Add the remaining onions, pine nuts, cinnamon, and allspice and sauté until onions are soft, about 2 minutes.

7. Spread onion and pine nut mixture evenly over first layer of meat in baking dish. Take remaining half of meat mixture and spread smoothly on top, using procedure in step 5.

8. Score top in diamond shapes with a knife dipped in cold water. Melt remaining 1½ tablespoons of butter and drizzle over top of the meat. Bake for approximately 40–45 minutes, or until gold brown.

Slow-Cooker Beef Braciole

NUTRITIONAL ANALYSIS (per serving)

Calories: **367**   Protein: **29g**   Carbohydrates: **25.93g**   Fat: **16g**   Saturated Fat: **5g**   Cholesterol: **69mg**   Sodium: **162mg**
Fiber: **5g**   PCF Ratio: **32-29-39**   Exchange Approx.: 3½ Very-Lean Meats, 2½ Fats, 3 Vegetables, 1 Starch

INGREDIENTS | SERVES 4

4 cups tomato sauce
1 tablespoon olive oil
¼ cup finely chopped onion
1 teaspoon finely chopped garlic
¼ cup finely chopped carrots
¼ cup finely chopped celery
2 slices whole-wheat bread, cubed
1 egg, lightly beaten
1 pound thinly sliced round beef, cut into 4 pieces

1. Place tomato sauce in a slow cooker and maintain at medium heat.

2. In a large nonstick skillet heat the olive oil. Add the onions, garlic, carrots, and celery and sauté until softened, about 5 minutes. Remove from heat.

3. Add the cubed bread and egg to sautéed vegetables and mix well.

4. Pound each piece of beef on both sides to flatten and tenderize. Each slice of meat should be about ¼" thick. Place approximately ½ cup of bread and vegetable stuffing down center of each meat slice and press in place. Starting at one end, roll meat up like a jelly roll and secure with 6" wooden skewer.

5. Place meat rolls in the tomato sauce. Set slow cooker on low setting and cook for at least 6 hours. (On low setting, the meat rolls can be left in slow cooker for 6–8 hours.) Remove wooden skewers before serving.

Soy and Ginger Flank Steak

NUTRITIONAL ANALYSIS (per serving)

Calories: 304   Protein: 29g   Carbohydrates: 1g   Fat: 19g   Saturated Fat: 7g   Cholesterol: 95mg   Sodium: 213mg
Fiber: 0g   PCF Ratio: 40-2-58   Exchange Approx.: 4 Lean Meats, 1½ Fats

INGREDIENTS | SERVES 4

1 pound lean London broil
1 tablespoon minced fresh ginger
2 teaspoons minced fresh garlic
1 tablespoon reduced-sodium soy sauce
3 tablespoons dry red wine
¼ teaspoon pepper
½ tablespoon olive oil

Slicing Meats Against the Grain

Certain cuts of meat such as flank steak, brisket, and London broil have a distinct grain (or line) of fibers running through them. If you slice with the grain, meat will seem tough and difficult to chew. These cuts of meat should always be thinly sliced across (or against) the grain so fibers are cut through and meats remain tender and easy to chew.

1. Place the meat, ginger, garlic, soy sauce, red wine, pepper, and olive oil in a shallow baking dish. Coat meat with marinade on both sides. Cover and refrigerate meat in marinade, turning meat once or twice during marinating so all marinade soaks into both sides of meat. Marinate the meat at least 3–4 hours.

2. Lightly oil a barbecue grill and preheat. Place marinated flank steak on grill. Grill steak, turning once, until done to your preference. Medium-rare will take approximately 12–15 minutes. Slice meat diagonally and against grain into thin slices.

Pork Lo Mein

NUTRITIONAL ANALYSIS (per serving)

Calories: **266** Protein: **23g** Carbohydrates: **25g** Fat: **8g** Saturated Fat: **2g** Cholesterol: **50mg** Sodium: **386mg** Fiber: **5g** PCF Ratio: **35-38-27** Exchange Approx.: **2½ Lean Meats, 1 Starch, 1 Vegetable**

INGREDIENTS | SERVES 4

1½ tablespoons reduced-sodium soy sauce

1 teaspoon fresh grated ginger

1 tablespoon rice vinegar

¼ teaspoon turmeric

¾ pound lean pork loin, cut into 1" cubes

½ tablespoon canola oil

½ cup sliced green onion

2 teaspoons minced garlic

2 cups shredded cabbage

1 cup snap peas, cut into 1" pieces

¼ teaspoon crushed red pepper

2 cups cooked whole-grain spaghetti

1 teaspoon sesame oil

1 teaspoon sesame seeds

1. Combine the soy sauce, ginger, rice vinegar, and turmeric in a bowl. Mix in cubed pork and set aside.

2. In a large skillet or wok, heat the canola oil and sauté the onion and garlic, for approximately 2 minutes. Add the meat and cook quickly until meat and onions are slightly browned, about 3–5 minutes.

3. Add in the cabbage and snap peas and continue to stir-fry for another 3–4 minutes. Sprinkle in the crushed red pepper.

4. When vegetables are crisp-tender, add cooked pasta, sesame oil, and sesame seeds. Toss lightly and serve.

Pork Roast with Caramelized Onions and Apples

NUTRITIONAL ANALYSIS (per serving)

Calories: 373   Protein: 31g   Carbohydrates: 8g   Fat: 23g   Saturated Fat: 9g   Cholesterol: 96mg   Sodium: 156mg
Fiber: 1g   PCF Ratio: 34-9-57   Exchange Approx.: 1 Vegetable, 4 Lean Meats, 2 Fats

INGREDIENTS | SERVES 6

2 pounds lean pork loin roast

Fresh ground pepper, to taste

½ tablespoon olive oil

½ tablespoon butter

2 cups chopped onion

1 tablespoon Marsala wine

⅓ cup low-sodium chicken broth

1 apple, peeled and chopped

1. Preheat the oven to 375°F.

2. Season the pork loin with pepper. Heat the olive oil in a large skillet and sear to brown all sides. Searing all sides takes 5–7 minutes.

3. Transfer roast to a 9" × 13" glass baking dish and place in oven for approximately 1 hour and 15 minutes.

4. While the pork is roasting, prepare the onions: In a large nonstick skillet, melt the butter and add the onions. Sauté onions until soft, approximately 2 minutes.

5. Add the wine, chicken broth, and apple. Continue cooking on low heat until onions are soft, brown in color, and have caramelized, approximately 20 minutes.

6. When roast has reached an internal temperature of 130°F, spoon the onions over top. Place a loose foil tent over the roast.

7. Remove roast from oven when an internal temperature of 145°F has been reached. (Temperature of roast will continue to rise as meat rests.) Keep roast loosely covered with foil and allow to stand for 10–15 minutes before slicing.

Fruited Pork Loin Roast Casserole

NUTRITIONAL ANALYSIS (per serving)

Calories: 170   Protein: 7g   Carbohydrates: 27g   Fat: 4g   Saturated Fat: 1g   Cholesterol: 19mg   Sodium: 32mg
Fiber: 3g   PCF Ratio: 17-63-20   Exchange Approx.: 1 Lean Meat, 1 Fruit, 1 Starch

INGREDIENTS | SERVES 4

4 small Yukon Gold potatoes, peeled and sliced

2 (2-ounce) pieces trimmed boneless pork loin, pounded flat

1 apple, peeled, cored, and sliced

4 apricot halves

1 tablespoon chopped red onion or shallot

⅛ cup apple cider or apple juice

Olive oil, to taste (optional)

Parmesan cheese, to taste (optional)

Salt and freshly ground pepper, to taste (optional)

Tip

To enhance the flavor of this dish, top with the optional ingredients when it's served. Just be sure to make the appropriate Exchange Approximations adjustments if you do.

1. Preheat the oven to 350°F (325°F if using a glass casserole dish). Treat casserole dish with nonstick spray.

2. Layer half of potato slices across bottom of dish; top with 1 piece of flattened pork loin. Arrange apple slices over the top of the loin. Place apricot halves on top of the apple. Sprinkle red onion over apricot and apples. Add second flattened pork loin; layer remaining potatoes atop loin. Drizzle apple cider over top of casserole.

3. Cover and bake for 45 minutes to 1 hour, or until potatoes are tender. Keep casserole covered and let sit for 10 minutes after removing from oven.

White Wine and Lemon Pork Roast

NUTRITIONAL ANALYSIS (per serving)

Calories: 172   Protein: 18g   Carbohydrates: 2g   Fat: 7g   Saturated Fat: 2g   Cholesterol: 50mg   Sodium: 47mg
Fiber: 0g   PCF Ratio: 53-5-42   Exchange Approx.: 3 Lean Meats

INGREDIENTS | SERVES 4

1 clove garlic, crushed

½ cup dry white wine

1 tablespoon lemon juice

1 teaspoon olive oil

1 tablespoon minced red onion or shallot

¼ teaspoon dried thyme

⅛ teaspoon ground black pepper

12 ounces pork loin roast

Marmalade Marinade

Combine 1 teaspoon Dijon or stone-ground mustard, 1 tablespoon Smucker's Low-Sugar Orange Marmalade, 1 clove crushed garlic, and ¼ teaspoon dried thyme leaves. Marinate and prepare a ½-pound (8-ounce) pork loin as you would the White Wine and Lemon Pork Roast. The Nutritional Analysis for a 2-ounce serving is: Calories: 89.52; Protein: 12.26g; Carbohydrates: 1.90g; Fat: 3.26g; Saturated Fat: 1.11g; Cholesterol: 33.45mg; Sodium: 43.66mg; Fiber: 0.09g; PCF Ratio: 57-9-34; Exchange Approximations: 2 Lean Meats.

1. Make the marinade by combining the garlic, white wine, lemon juice, olive oil, red onion, thyme, and black pepper in heavy, freezer-style plastic bag.

2. Add the roast to the bag and marinate in the refrigerator for 1 hour or overnight, according to taste. (Note: Pork loin is already tender, so you're marinating the meat to impart the flavors only.)

3. Preheat the oven to 350°F.

4. Remove the meat from marinade and put on nonstick spray–treated roasting rack in a roasting pan. Roast for 20–30 minutes, or until meat thermometer reads 150°F–170°F, depending on how well done you prefer it.

Balsamic Venison Pot Roast

NUTRITIONAL ANALYSIS (per serving)

Calories: **188**   Protein: **28g**   Carbohydrates: **6g**   Fat: **6g**   Saturated Fat: **2g**   Cholesterol: **70mg**   Sodium: **75mg**
Fiber: **1g**   PCF Ratio: **60-13-28**   Exchange Approx.: **4 Very-Lean Meats, ½ Fat**

INGREDIENTS | SERVES 8

2½ tablespoons all-purpose flour

2 teaspoons paprika

2-pound venison roast

1½ tablespoons olive oil

14 ounces low-sodium beef broth

½ cup chopped onion

2 tablespoons dried onion flakes

⅓ cup balsamic vinegar

⅛ teaspoon Worcestershire sauce

1 teaspoon sugar

Recipe Adaptation

This recipe also works well cooked in a slow cooker for 6–8 hours, until tender. Slow cookers with a ceramic interior maintain low temperatures better than those with a metal cooking surface.

1. On a large plate, mix the flour and paprika together.

2. Dredge the venison in the flour mixture and completely coat with flour.

3. Heat oil in a Dutch oven or deep skillet. Add the roast and brown on all sides, about 5–7 minutes to brown all sides.

4. Add the beef broth, onion, onion flakes, balsamic vinegar, Worcestershire sauce, and sugar to the skillet. Bring to a quick boil.

5. Reduce heat to low. Cover and cook over low heat for 2–3 hours, or until venison is tender and cuts easily. Serve with whole-grain noodles.

Venison Pepper Steak

NUTRITIONAL ANALYSIS (per serving)

Calories: **237**   Protein: **26g**   Carbohydrates: **12g**   Fat: **9g**   Saturated Fat: **3g**   Cholesterol: **39mg**   Sodium: **344mg**
Fiber: **2g**   PCF Ratio: **44-20-36**   Exchange Approx.: **3½ Very-Lean Meats, 2 Vegetables, 1½ Fats**

INGREDIENTS | SERVES 4

1 pound venison loin

2 tablespoons reduced-sodium soy sauce

1 clove garlic

1½ teaspoons ginger, grated

1 tablespoon canola oil

1 cup onion, thinly sliced

1 cup green or red peppers, cut into ½" strips

½ cup thinly sliced celery

1 tablespoon cornstarch

1 cup water

1½ cups chopped tomatoes

1. Cut meat across grain into ¼" strips.

2. In a small bowl, combine the soy sauce, garlic, and ginger. Add the sliced meat and mix well. Set aside.

3. Heat the canola oil in large wok or skillet. Add meat and cook for 2–3 minutes over high heat. Cover, reduce heat, and simmer for 15 minutes.

4. Add the onions, peppers, and celery to the meat. Cover and cook on low heat for 15 minutes, or until sliced meat is tender.

5. In small bowl, mix the cornstarch with the water. Add to the meat. Cook for 5 minutes, or until the sauce thickens slightly. Add tomatoes and heat through.

Whole-Grain Additions

Instead of serving white rice, substitute brown rice or quinoa mixed with sautéed vegetables with this dish.

Slow-Cooker Venison and Vegetable Pot Roast

NUTRITIONAL ANALYSIS (per serving)

Calories: 309   Protein: 27g   Carbohydrates: 28g   Fat: 10g   Saturated Fat: 3g   Cholesterol: 39mg   Sodium: 237mg
Fiber: 4g   PCF Ratio: 35-36-28   Exchange Approx.: 3½ Very-Lean Meats, 1 Starch, 3 Vegetables, 1½ Fats

INGREDIENTS | SERVES 4

1 pound venison roast

1 tablespoon all-purpose flour

1 tablespoon olive oil

1 tablespoon instant brown gravy mix

1 teaspoon Worcestershire sauce

1 cup chopped onions

½ pound potatoes, cut into 1" pieces

1 cup carrots, cut into 1" pieces

1 cup chopped celery

½ cup crushed tomato

½ teaspoon dried thyme leaves

1. Dredge roast in flour. Heat olive oil in large skillet; sear roast until browned on all sides, about 5–7 minutes. Put roast in slow cooker.

2. Sprinkle the instant gravy mix and Worcestershire sauce over top of roast. Place the onions, potatoes, carrots, and celery around roast. Spoon crushed tomatoes evenly around vegetables. Sprinkle thyme over meat and vegetables.

3. Cook in slow cooker on low setting for 6–8 hours.

Variation

You can also use ⅓ cup water and 2 tablespoons red wine for the liquid instead of crushed tomatoes.

CHAPTER 10

Poultry Dishes

Chicken Broth: Easy Slow-Cooker Method

NUTRITIONAL ANALYSIS (per serving)

Calories: 67   Protein: 9g   Carbohydrates: 0g   Fat: 3g   Saturated Fat: 1g   Cholesterol: 24mg   Sodium: 22mg
Fiber: 0g   PCF Ratio: 53-0-47   Exchange Approx.: ½ Very-Lean Meat, ½ Lean Meat

INGREDIENTS	YIELDS ABOUT 4 CUPS; SERVING SIZE: ½ CUP

1 small onion, chopped

2 carrots, peeled and chopped

2 celery stalks and leaves, chopped

1 bay leaf

4 sprigs parsley

6 black peppercorns

¼ cup dry white wine

2 pounds chicken pieces, skin removed

4½ cups water

Reduced Broth

Reducing broth is the act of boiling it to decrease the amount of water so you're left with a richer broth. Boiling nonfat, canned chicken broth won't reduce it as a home-made broth would. The broth from this recipe will be richer than what most recipes call for, so unless you need reduced broth, thin it with water as needed. Assuming you remove the fat from the broth, it will be a Free Exchange.

1. Add all the ingredients except water to a slow cooker. The chicken pieces and vegetables should be loosely layered and fill no more than ¾ of slow cooker.

2. Add enough water to just cover ingredients. Cover the slow cooker. Set slow cooker to high until the mixture almost reaches a boil, then reduce heat to low. Allow to simmer overnight or up to 16 hours, checking occasionally and adding more water, if necessary.

3. Remove chicken pieces and drain on paper towels to absorb any fat. Allow to cool; remove meat from bones. Strain vegetables from broth and discard. (You don't want to eat vegetables cooked directly with chicken because they will have absorbed too much of the residue fat.)

4. Put broth in a covered container and refrigerate for several hours or overnight, allowing the fat to congeal on top. Remove hardened fat and discard.

5. To separate broth into small amounts for use when you steam vegetables or potatoes, fill up an ice cube tray with stock. Let freeze, then remove cubes from tray and store in labeled freezer bag. Common ice cube trays allow for ⅛ cup or 2 tablespoons of liquid per section.

Oven-Fried Chicken Thighs

NUTRITIONAL ANALYSIS (per serving, no oil)

Calories: 74   Protein: 9g   Carbohydrates: 5g   Fat: 2g   Saturated Fat: 1g   Cholesterol: 34mg   Sodium: 331mg
Fiber: 0g   PCF Ratio: 53-26-21   Exchange Approx.: 2 Very-Lean Meats

INGREDIENTS | SERVES 4

4 chicken thighs, skin removed

1 tablespoon unbleached, white all-purpose flour

1 large egg white

½ teaspoon sea salt

½ teaspoon olive oil (optional; see Comparison Analysis for using olive oil)

1 tablespoon rice flour

1 tablespoon cornmeal

If You Use Oil . . .

Comparison Analysis (with olive oil): Calories: 78.53; Protein: 9.46g; Carbohydrates: 4.65g; Fat: 2.27g; Saturated Fat: 0.50g; Cholesterol: 34.03mg; Sodium: 331.03mg; Fiber: 0.06g; PCF Ratio: 49-24-27; Exchange Approx.: 2 Lean Meats.

1. Preheat the oven to 350°F. Spray a baking sheet with nonstick cooking spray.

2. Rinse and dry chicken thighs. Put white flour on plate.

3. In a small, shallow bowl, whip the egg white with the sea salt. Add olive oil if using and mix well.

4. Put rice flour and cornmeal on another plate and mix together.

5. Roll each chicken thigh in the white flour, then dip it into the egg mixture, and then roll it in rice flour mixture.

6. Place thighs on rack so they aren't touching. Bake for 35–45 minutes, until meat juices run clear.

Another Healthy "Fried" Chicken

NUTRITIONAL ANALYSIS (per serving)

Calories: **118** Protein: **19g** Carbohydrates: **5g** Fat: **2g** Saturated Fat: **1g** Cholesterol: **44mg** Sodium: **91mg** Fiber: **0g** PCF Ratio: **66-18-16** Exchange Approx.: **2 Very-Lean Meats, ½ Starch**

INGREDIENTS | SERVES 4

10 ounces raw boneless, skinless chicken breasts (fat trimmed off)

½ cup nonfat plain yogurt

½ cup bread crumbs

1 teaspoon garlic powder

1 teaspoon paprika

¼ teaspoon dried thyme

Chicken Fat Facts

When faced with the decision of whether to have chicken with or without the skin, consider that ½ pound of skinless chicken breast has 9g of fat; ½ pound with the skin on has 38g!

1. Preheat the oven to 350°F. Prepare a baking pan with nonstick cooking spray.

2. Cut the chicken breast into 4 equal pieces. Marinate chicken pieces in the yogurt for several minutes.

3. On a plate, mix together the bread crumbs, garlic, paprika, and thyme.

4. Dredge the chicken in the crumb mixture. Arrange on the prepared pan and bake for 20 minutes. To give chicken a deep golden color, place pan under broiler last 5 minutes of cooking. Watch closely to ensure chicken "crust" doesn't burn.

Buttermilk Ranch Chicken Salad

NUTRITIONAL ANALYSIS (per serving)

Calories: 147   Protein: 18g   Carbohydrates: 11g   Fat: 4g   Saturated Fat: 1g   Cholesterol: 33mg   Sodium: 184mg
Fiber: 2g   PCF Ratio: 49-29-22   Exchange Approx.: 2 Very-Lean Meats, ½ Vegetable, 1 Free Vegetable, ½ Skim Milk

INGREDIENTS | SERVES 4

1 cup chopped cooked chicken breast

½ cup sliced cucumber

½ cup chopped celery

½ cup sliced carrots

1 tablespoon real mayonnaise

3 tablespoons nonfat plain yogurt

½ cup nonfat cottage cheese

½ teaspoon cider vinegar

1 teaspoon brown sugar

1 teaspoon Dijon mustard

½ cup buttermilk

2 tablespoons dried parsley

1 clove garlic, minced

2 tablespoons grated Parmesan cheese

¼ teaspoon sea salt (optional)

¼ teaspoon freshly ground pepper (optional)

4 cups salad greens

½ cup red onion slices

Fresh parsley for garnish (optional)

1. In a large bowl combine the chicken, cucumber, celery, and carrots.

2. In a blender or food processor, combine the mayonnaise, yogurt, cottage cheese, vinegar, brown sugar, mustard, buttermilk, parsley, garlic, cheese, salt, and pepper and process until smooth. Pour over the chicken mixture in the bowl. Chill for at least 2 hours.

3. To serve, arrange 1 cup of salad greens on each of 4 serving plates. Top each salad with an equal amount of chicken salad. Garnish with red onion slices and fresh parsley, if desired.

Get More Mileage from Your Meals

Leftover chicken salad makes great sandwiches. Put it between two slices of bread with lots of lettuce for a quick lunch. The lettuce helps keep the bread from getting soggy if the sandwich is to go.

Pineapple-Orange Grilled Chicken Breasts

NUTRITIONAL ANALYSIS (per serving)

Calories: **165**   Protein: **27g**   Carbohydrates: **10g**   Fat: **2g**   Saturated Fat: **0g**   Cholesterol: **58.40mg**   Sodium: **75mg**
Fiber: **0g**   PCF Ratio: **67-25-9**   Exchange Approx.: **3½ Lean Meats, ½ Fruit**

INGREDIENTS | SERVES 4

6 ounces pineapple juice

4 ounces orange juice

¼ cup cider vinegar

1 tablespoon fresh tarragon, chopped

½ tablespoon fresh rosemary

1 pound boneless chicken breast, skinned and cut into 4 pieces

1. About 3–4 hours before you are ready to grill, make the marinade: In a large shallow dish, combine the pineapple juice, orange juice, vinegar, tarragon, and rosemary.

2. Add the raw chicken breasts to the marinade. Cover and refrigerate for 3–4 hours. Turn pieces of chicken over during marinade process to cover with marinade.

3. Heat the grill to medium-high.

4. Place the chicken on the grill. Grill for approximately 7–10 minutes on each side, until chicken is cooked through.

Herbed Chicken and Brown Rice Dinner

NUTRITIONAL ANALYSIS (per serving)

Calories: 300   Protein: 33g   Carbohydrates: 26g   Fat: 6g   Saturated Fat: 1g   Cholesterol: 75mg   Sodium: 112mg
Fiber: 3g   PCF Ratio: 45-36-19   Exchange Approx.: 1½ Starches, 2 Very-Lean Meats, 2 Lean Meats

INGREDIENTS | SERVES 4

1 tablespoon canola oil

4 (4-ounce) boneless chicken breast pieces, skin removed

¾ teaspoon garlic powder

¾ teaspoon dried rosemary

1 (10½-ounce) can low-fat, reduced-sodium chicken broth

⅓ cup water

2 cups uncooked instant brown rice

1. Heat oil in a large nonstick skillet over medium-high. Add the chicken and sprinkle it with half the garlic powder and half the crushed rosemary. Cover and cook for 4 minutes on each side, or until cooked through. Remove chicken from skillet and set aside.

2. Add broth and water to the skillet. Stir to deglaze pan and bring to a boil. Stir in rice and remaining garlic powder and rosemary.

3. Top with the chicken and cover. Cook on low heat for 5 minutes.

4. Remove from heat and let stand, covered, for 5 minutes.

Walnut Chicken

NUTRITIONAL ANALYSIS (per serving)

Calories: **159**   Protein: **18g**   Carbohydrates: **1g**   Fat: **9g**   Saturated Fat: **1g**   Cholesterol: **44mg**   Sodium: **51mg**
Fiber: **1g**   PCF Ratio: **47-3-51**   Exchange Approx.: **2 Very-Lean Meats, 1½ Fats**

INGREDIENTS | SERVES 4

¾ pound (12 ounces) raw boneless, skinless chicken breast

1 teaspoon sherry

1 egg white

2 teaspoons peanut oil

2 drops toasted sesame oil (optional)

⅓ cup ground walnuts

1. Preheat the oven to 350°F.

2. Cut the chicken into bite-sized pieces. Sprinkle the pieces with sherry and set aside.

3. In a small bowl, beat the egg white and oils until frothy.

4. Fold chicken pieces into the egg mixture, then roll the pieces individually in chopped walnuts.

5. Arrange the chicken pieces on a baking sheet treated with nonstick cooking spray. Bake for 10–15 minutes, or until walnuts are lightly browned and chicken juices run clear. (Walnuts make the fat ratio of this dish high, so serve it with steamed vegetables and rice to bring the ratios into balance.)

Easy Chicken Paprikash

NUTRITIONAL ANALYSIS (per serving, equal amounts of light and dark meat chicken)

Calories: 376   Protein: 22g   Carbohydrates: 58g   Fat: 6g   Saturated Fat: 2g   Cholesterol: 78mg   Sodium: 135mg
Fiber: 4g   PCF Ratio: 23-62-15   Exchange Approx.: ½ Very-Lean Meat, ½ Lean Meat, 2½ Starches, 1 Vegetable, 1 Skim Milk

INGREDIENTS | SERVES 4

1 recipe Condensed Cream of Chicken Soup (see Chapter 12)

½ cup skim milk

2 teaspoons sweet paprika

⅛ teaspoon ground red pepper (optional)

¼ pound (4 ounces) chopped cooked boneless, skinless chicken

1½ cups sliced steamed mushrooms

½ cup diced steamed onion

½ cup nonfat plain yogurt

4 cups cooked medium-sized egg noodles

1. In a saucepan, combine the soup, skim milk, paprika, and pepper (if using), and whisk until well mixed. Bring to a boil over medium heat, stirring occasionally.

2. Reduce heat to low and stir in chicken, mushrooms, and onion. Cook until chicken and vegetables are heated through, about 10 minutes. Stir in yogurt.

3. To serve, put 1 cup of warm, cooked noodles on each of 4 plates. Top each portion with an equal amount of chicken mixture. Garnish by sprinkling with additional paprika, if desired.

For Best Results . . .

Mock condensed soup recipes are used in the dishes in this book so that you know the accurate Nutritional Analysis information. In all cases, you can substitute commercial canned condensed soups; however, be sure to use the lower fat and sodium varieties.

Chicken and Broccoli Casserole

NUTRITIONAL ANALYSIS (per serving)

Calories: 328   Protein: 26g   Carbohydrates: 20g   Fat: 17g   Saturated Fat: 6g   Cholesterol: 67mg   Sodium: 254mg
Fiber: 3g   PCF Ratio: 31-24-45   Exchange Approx.: 1 Very-Lean Meat, 1 Lean Meat, ½ High-Fat Meat, 1 Fat, 1 Vegetable, 1 Skim Milk, ½ Starch

INGREDIENTS | SERVES 4

2 cups broccoli

½ pound (8 ounces) cooked chopped chicken

½ cup skim milk

⅛ cup (2 tablespoons) real mayonnaise

¼ teaspoon curry powder

1 recipe Condensed Cream of Chicken Soup (see Chapter 12)

1 tablespoon lemon juice

½ cup (2 ounces) grated Cheddar cheese

½ cup bread crumbs

1 teaspoon melted butter

1 teaspoon olive oil

1. Preheat the oven to 350°F. Treat an 11" × 7" casserole dish with nonstick spray.

2. Steam broccoli until tender, then drain.

3. Spread out chicken on the bottom of dish. Cover with the steamed broccoli.

4. In a medium bowl, combine the milk, mayonnaise, curry powder, soup, and lemon juice. Pour mixture over broccoli.

5. In a small bowl, mix together the cheese, bread crumbs, butter, and oil. Sprinkle over the top of the casserole. Bake for 30 minutes.

Chicken and Green Bean Stovetop Casserole

NUTRITIONAL ANALYSIS (per serving)

Calories: 305 Protein: 23 Carbohydrates: 36g Fat: 8g Saturated Fat: 2g Cholesterol: 48mg Sodium: 101mg
Fiber: 6g PCF Ratio: 30-46-24 Exchange Approx.: 1 Very-Lean Meat, 1 Lean Meat, 1 Vegetable, 1 Starch, 1 Skim Milk

INGREDIENTS | SERVES 4

1 recipe Condensed Cream of Chicken Soup (see Chapter 12)

¼ cup skim milk

2 teaspoons Worcestershire sauce (recipe for homemade in Chapter 16)

1 teaspoon real mayonnaise

½ teaspoon onion powder

¼ teaspoon garlic powder

¼ teaspoon ground black pepper

1 (4-ounce) can sliced water chestnuts, drained

2½ cups frozen green beans, thawed

1 cup sliced mushrooms, steamed

½ pound (8 ounces) cooked chopped chicken

1⅓ cups cooked brown long-grain rice

Veggie Filler

Steamed mushrooms are a low-calorie way to add flavor to a dish and "stretch" the meat. If you don't like mushrooms, you can substitute an equal amount of other low-calorie steamed vegetables like red and green peppers and not significantly affect the total calories in a recipe.

1. In a saucepan, combine the soup, milk, Worcestershire, mayonnaise, onion powder, garlic powder, and pepper and bring to a boil.

2. Reduce heat, add the water chestnuts, green beans, mushrooms, and chicken. Simmer until vegetables and chicken are heated through, about 10 minutes. Serve over rice.

Chicken and Asparagus in White Wine Sauce

NUTRITIONAL ANALYSIS (per serving)

Calories: 186   Protein: 21g   Carbohydrates: 7g   Fat: 8g   Saturated Fat: 2g   Cholesterol: 51mg   Sodium: 57mg
Fiber: 2g   PCF Ratio: 46-16-38   Exchange Approx.: 2½ Very-Lean Meats, 1½ Vegetables, 1 Fat

INGREDIENTS | SERVES 4

4 boneless, skinless chicken breast halves

½ tablespoon butter

1 tablespoon olive oil

1 teaspoon garlic, finely chopped

½ cup onion, finely chopped

10 ounces asparagus spears, cut diagonally in 2" pieces

½ pound mushrooms

¼ cup dry white wine

¼ cup water

1 tablespoon chopped parsley

Salt and pepper, to taste

1. Pound the chicken pieces to ¼" thickness.

2. Melt butter and olive oil in a large skillet over medium heat. Add chopped garlic and onions and sauté for 1–2 minutes.

3. Add chicken and cook for 5 minutes, or until the chicken is brown on both sides. Remove chicken and set aside.

4. Add the asparagus and mushrooms to skillet. Cook for 2–3 minutes.

5. Return the chicken to skillet; add white wine and water. Bring to a quick boil. Boil for 2 minutes to reduce the liquid.

6. Reduce heat. Cover and simmer for 3 minutes, or until the chicken and vegetables are tender. Add chopped parsley, salt, and pepper to taste, and serve.

Chicken Kalamata

NUTRITIONAL ANALYSIS (per serving)

Calories: **311**   Protein: **31g**   Carbohydrates: **25g**   Fat: **11g**   Saturated Fat: **2g**   Cholesterol: **66mg**   Sodium: **787mg**
Fiber: **6g**   PCF Ratio: **38-31-31**   Exchange Approx.: **4 Lean Meats, 2 Vegetables, 1 Starch, 2 Fats**

INGREDIENTS | SERVES 4

2 tablespoons olive oil
1 cup chopped onion
1 teaspoon minced garlic
1½ cups chopped green peppers
1 pound boneless, skinless chicken breast, cut into 4 pieces
2 cups diced tomatoes
1 teaspoon oregano
½ cup pitted, chopped kalamata olives

1. Heat the olive oil over medium heat in a large skillet. Add the onions, garlic, and peppers and sauté for about 5 minutes until the onions are translucent.

2. Add the chicken pieces. Cook for about 5 minutes each side until lightly brown.

3. Add the tomatoes and oregano. Reduce heat and simmer for 20 minutes.

4. Add the olives and simmer for an additional 10 minutes before serving.

Are Olives Counted as a Fruit or Vegetable?

The short answer is: Neither! Even though olives are a fruit that grows on trees, their flesh is filled with a significant amount of oil and therefore is counted as a fat. Nine black olives or ten green olives equals 1 Fat Serving. The health benefits of olives (and olive oil) comes from the monounsaturated fats they contain. Olives are usually cured in a brine, salt, or olive oil, so if you must watch your salt intake, be careful how many you eat.

Chicken Breasts in Balsamic Vinegar Sauce

NUTRITIONAL ANALYSIS (per serving)

Calories: 200   Protein: 28g   Carbohydrates: 2g   Fat: 8g   Saturated Fat: 3g   Cholesterol: 73mg   Sodium: 381mg
Fiber: 0g   PCF Ratio: 58-4-38   Exchange Approx.: 4 Lean Meats, 1½ Fats

INGREDIENTS | SERVES 4

1 pound boneless, skinless chicken breasts, cut into 4 pieces

Pinch salt

¼ teaspoon pepper

1 tablespoon butter

1 tablespoon olive oil

¼ cup red onion, chopped

2 teaspoons finely chopped garlic

3 tablespoons balsamic vinegar

1½ cups low-sodium chicken broth

1 teaspoon oregano

1. Sprinkle the chicken with salt and pepper.

2. Heat butter and olive oil in a large skillet over medium heat. Add the chicken and cook until browned, about 5 minutes each side.

3. Reduce heat and cook for 12 minutes. Transfer to a platter, cover, and keep warm.

4. Add the red onions and garlic to the skillet. Sauté over medium heat for 3 minutes, scraping up the browned bits.

5. Add the balsamic vinegar and bring to a boil. Boil for 3 minutes, or until reduced to a glaze, stirring constantly.

6. Add the chicken broth. Boil until reduced to about ¾ cup liquid. Remove sauce from heat and add the chopped oregano. Spoon sauce over chicken and serve immediately.

Chicken Thighs Cacciatore

NUTRITIONAL ANALYSIS (per serving)

Calories: **370**   Protein: **19g**   Carbohydrates: **48g**   Fat: **9g**   Saturated Fat: **2g**   Cholesterol: **39mg**   Sodium: **166mg**
Fiber: **4g**   PCF Ratio: **21-55-24**   Exchange Approx.: **1½ Lean Meats, 2½ Starches, 1 Fat, 1 Vegetable**

INGREDIENTS | SERVES 4

2 teaspoons olive oil
½ cup chopped onion
2 cloves garlic, minced
4 chicken thighs, skin removed
½ cup dry red wine
1 (14½-ounce) can unsalted diced tomatoes, undrained
1 teaspoon dried parsley
½ teaspoon dried oregano
¼ teaspoon pepper
⅛ teaspoon sugar
¼ cup grated Parmesan cheese
4 cups cooked spaghetti
2 teaspoons extra-virgin olive oil

For Cheese Lovers!

Indulge your love of extra cheese and still have a main dish that's under 400 calories. Prepare Chicken Thighs Cacciatore according to recipe instructions. Top each portion with 1 tablespoon freshly grated Parmesan cheese. With cheese, analysis is: Calories: 398.22; Protein: 21.39g; Carbohydrates: 48.43g; Fat: 11.15g; Saturated Fat: 3.62g; Cholesterol: 43.87mg; Sodium: 282.14mg; Fiber: 3.81g; PCF Ratio: 23-51-26; Exchange Approx.: 2 Lean Meats, 2½ Starches, 1 Fat, 1 Vegetable.

1. Heat a deep, nonstick skillet over medium-high heat and add 2 teaspoons olive oil. Add the onion and sauté until transparent, approximately 2–3 minutes.

2. Add the garlic and chicken thighs and sauté for 3 minutes on each side, or until lightly browned. Remove thighs from pan.

3. Add the wine, tomatoes and juices, parsley, oregano, pepper, and sugar to the pan. Stir well and bring to a boil.

4. Add the chicken back to pan. Sprinkle Parmesan cheese over top. Cover, reduce heat, and simmer for 10 minutes.

5. Uncover and simmer for 10 more minutes.

6. To serve, put 1 cup of cooked pasta on each of 4 plates. Top each serving with a chicken thigh. Divide sauce between dishes. Drizzle ½ teaspoon extra-virgin olive oil over top of each dish and serve.

Chicken with Portobello Mushrooms and Roasted Garlic

INGREDIENTS | SERVES 4

1 tablespoon olive oil

4 boneless, skinless chicken breasts

1 cup reduced-sodium chicken broth

1 bulb garlic, dry-roasted (see sidebar) and mashed into paste

1 tablespoon butter

2 cups Portobello mushrooms, chopped

½ teaspoon thyme

2 tablespoons crumbled feta cheese

Dry-Roasted Garlic

To dry-roast garlic: Preheat oven to 350°F; lightly spray small, covered baking dish with nonstick spray. Slice off ½" from top of each garlic head; rub off any loose skins, being careful not to separate cloves. Place in baking dish, cut-side up (if roasting more than 1 head, arrange in dish so they don't touch). Cover and bake until the garlic cloves are very tender when pierced, about 30–45 minutes. Roasted garlic heads will keep in refrigerator 2–3 days.

1. Heat the olive oil in a large nonstick skillet over medium heat. Brown the chicken breasts on both sides, about 5 minutes per side.

2. Add the chicken broth and roasted garlic paste to pan. Cover and simmer on low for 10 minutes.

3. Meanwhile, in a separate, smaller saucepan, sauté the mushrooms and thyme in the butter. Simmer for 2 minutes.

4. Add the mushrooms and thyme mixture to the chicken and simmer for an additional 2 minutes.

5. When serving, top each chicken breast with 1½ teaspoons feta cheese and pour sauce over the top.

Chipotle Chicken Wrap

NUTRITIONAL ANALYSIS (per serving)

Calories: **284**   Protein: **24g**   Carbohydrates: **28g**   Fat: **8g**   Saturated Fat: **2g**   Cholesterol: **40mg**   Sodium: **415mg**
Fiber: **2g**   PCF Ratio: **35-41-25**   Exchange Approx.: **2 Starches, ½ Vegetable, 3 Lean Meats**

INGREDIENTS | SERVES 4

12 ounces boneless, skinless chicken breast
1 tablespoon lime juice
1 tablespoon olive oil
1 teaspoon chipotle seasoning
⅛ teaspoon fresh ground pepper
4 whole-wheat tortillas
½ cup jarred salsa
1 cup chopped lettuce

What Is Chipotle?

A chipotle (chee-POTE-lay) is a smoke-dried jalapeño chili used in Mexican or Tex-Mex dishes. You can purchase dried chipotle peppers or a seasoning mix with chipotle peppers added. Mrs. Dash has a Southwest Chipotle Seasoning blend that is salt-free!

1. Cut the chicken into ½" strips. Place the chicken, lime juice, olive oil, chipotle seasoning, and pepper in a dish and mix well. Cover and allow chicken to marinate for 1 hour.

2. Heat outdoor grill. Wrap tortillas in aluminum foil and place on top rack. Cook chicken for 7–9 minutes until done, turning strips once during cooking.

3. When ready to make wraps, place chicken strips in center of each heated tortilla, add 2 tablespoons salsa to each, top with chopped lettuce, and wrap.

Stovetop Grilled Turkey Breast

NUTRITIONAL ANALYSIS (per serving)

Calories: 207   Protein: 31g   Carbohydrates: 2g   Fat: 8g   Saturated Fat: 2g   Cholesterol: 85mg   Sodium: 68mg
Fiber: 0g   PCF Ratio: 62-3-35   Exchange Approx.: 4 Very-Lean Meats, ½ Fat

INGREDIENTS | SERVES 4

1 teaspoon cider vinegar

1 teaspoon garlic powder

1 teaspoon Dijon mustard

1 teaspoon brown sugar

¼ teaspoon black pepper

2 teaspoons olive oil

4 (4-ounce) turkey breast cutlets

Tip

Cutlets prepared this way tend to cook faster than on an outdoor grill. If using an indoor grill that cooks both sides at once, allow 4–5 minutes total cooking time. You can also use a well-seasoned cast-iron skillet instead of a grill pan; however, you may need to introduce more oil to the pan to prevent the cutlets from sticking. Cooking time will be the same as with a grill pan. Be sure to adjust the Fat Exchange, if necessary.

1. In a medium bowl, combine the vinegar, garlic powder, mustard, brown sugar, and black pepper. Slowly whisk in olive oil to thoroughly combine and make a thin paste.

2. Rinse turkey cutlets and dry thoroughly on paper towels. If necessary to ensure a uniform thickness, put between sheets of plastic wrap and pound to flatten.

3. Pour paste into heavy-duty freezer-style resealable plastic bag. Add cutlets, moving around in mixture to coat all sides. Seal bag, carefully squeezing out as much air as possible. Refrigerate to allow turkey to marinate for at least 1 hour, or as long as overnight.

4. Place nonstick hard-anodized stovetop grill pan over high heat. When pan is heated thoroughly, add the cutlets. Lower heat to medium-high and cook the cutlets for 3 minutes on the first side. Use tongs to turn and cook for another 3 minutes, or until juices run clean.

Turkey Mushroom Burgers

NUTRITIONAL ANALYSIS (per serving)

Calories: **100**   Protein: **15g**   Carbohydrates: **3g**   Fat: **3g**   Saturated Fat: **1g**   Cholesterol: **34mg**   Sodium: **36mg**
Fiber: **1g**   PCF Ratio: **60-10-30**   Exchange Approx.: **1 Lean Meat, 1 Vegetable, ½ Fat**

INGREDIENTS | **YIELDS 8 LARGE BURGERS**

1-pound turkey breast
1 pound fresh button mushrooms
1 tablespoon olive oil
1 teaspoon butter
1 clove garlic, minced
1 tablespoon green onion, chopped
¼ teaspoon dried thyme
¼ teaspoon dried oregano
¼ teaspoon freshly ground black pepper
Cayenne pepper or dried red pepper flakes, to taste (optional)

1. Cut turkey into even pieces about 1" square. Place pieces in the freezer for 10 minutes, or long enough to allow turkey to become somewhat firm.

2. In a covered microwave-safe container, microwave the mushrooms on high for 3–4 minutes, or until they begin to soften and sweat. Set aside to cool slightly.

3. Process the turkey in a food processor until ground, scraping down sides of bowl as necessary.

4. Add the oil, butter, garlic, onion, and mushrooms (and any resulting liquid from the mushrooms) to the food processor. Process until the mushrooms are ground, scraping down sides of bowl as necessary.

5. Add the remaining ingredients and pulse until mixed. Shape into 8 equal-sized patties. Cooking times will vary according to method used and how thick burgers are.

Turkey Marsala with Fresh Peas

NUTRITIONAL ANALYSIS (per serving)

Calories: **278**   Protein: **30g**   Carbohydrates: **14g**   Fat: **7g**   Saturated Fat: **3g**   Cholesterol: **78mg**   Sodium: **208mg**
Fiber: **2g**   PCF Ratio: **50-24-27**   Exchange Approx.: **4 Very-Lean Meats, ½ Starch, ½ Vegetable, 1 Fat**

INGREDIENTS | SERVES 4

¼ cup all-purpose flour

¼ teaspoon salt

¼ teaspoon pepper

½ teaspoon paprika

1 pound raw turkey breast cutlets, sliced ¼" thick

1 tablespoon olive oil

1 tablespoon butter

½ cup onion, thinly sliced

½ cup Marsala wine

½ cup fresh or frozen peas

Quick Tip

It's easy to prepare quick and healthy meals if you keep skinless, boneless chicken or turkey in the freezer. If you use an indoor grill, you don't even need to thaw them first. You can prepare a quick sauce or glaze in the time it takes for the chicken or turkey to cook.

1. In a plastic zip-top bag, mix together the flour, salt, pepper, and paprika. Place turkey cutlets in a plastic bag and shake to coat cutlets with flour.

2. Heat the olive oil and butter in a large skillet. Add the onions and sauté for about 5 minutes, until browned.

3. Add the coated turkey cutlets. Brown on both sides, approximately 7–8 minutes on each side.

4. Add the Marsala to pan, stirring well to combine. Bring to a boil and reduce heat. Turn cutlets to coat both sides.

5. Add peas and continue to cook, stirring, for another 2–3 minutes. Serve.

Spicy Grilled Turkey Burgers

NUTRITIONAL ANALYSIS (per serving)

Calories: 176   Protein: 26g   Carbohydrates: 5g   Fat: 5g   Saturated Fat: 2g   Cholesterol: 125mg   Sodium: 155mg
Fiber: 0g   PCF Ratio: 63-12-25   Exchange Approx.: 3½ Very-Lean Meats, 1 Fat

INGREDIENTS | SERVES 4

1 pound ground turkey

¼ cup bread crumbs

1 tablespoon Cajun Blend seasoning (see Chapter 17) or commercial salt-free blend

1 egg

1 tablespoon fresh cilantro, finely chopped

2 teaspoons jalapeño pepper, minced

Nonstick cooking spray

1. In a large bowl, combine all the ingredients well. Shape the mixture into 4 patties.

2. Spray a grill with nonstick cooking spray. Grill burgers for approximately 6 minutes on each side, or until cooked through.

Proper Poultry and Meat Handling

Be sure to wash any utensil that comes in contact with raw poultry in hot, soapy water and rinse well. This includes washing any utensil each time it's used to baste grilling, roasting, or baking poultry.

Turkey Chili

NUTRITIONAL ANALYSIS (per serving)

Calories: 281 Protein: 26g Carbohydrates: 38g Fat: 4g Saturated Fat: 1g Cholesterol: 49mg Sodium: 347mg
Fiber: 11g PCF Ratio: 35-52-13 Exchange Approx.: 2 Starches, 2 Vegetables, 3 Very-Lean Meats, 1½ Fats

INGREDIENTS | SERVES 6

1 pound ground turkey
1 cup chopped onions
½ cup chopped green pepper
2 teaspoons garlic, finely chopped
2 (28-ounce) cans crushed tomatoes
1 cup canned black beans, drained
1 cup canned red kidney beans, drained
3 tablespoons chili powder
1 tablespoon ground cumin
1 teaspoon crushed red pepper
Dash Tabasco

1. Brown the ground turkey in a large nonstick pot over medium-high heat.

2. Drain off any fat and then add the chopped onion, green pepper, and garlic. Continue cooking until the onion is translucent, about 5 minutes.

3. Add the remaining ingredients and bring to a slow boil.

4. Reduce heat, cover, and let simmer for at least 2–3 hours before serving.

Turkey Kielbasa with Red Beans and Rice

NUTRITIONAL ANALYSIS (per serving)

Calories: 297 Protein: 15g Carbohydrates: 41g Fat: 9g Saturated Fat: 3g Cholesterol: 32mg Sodium: 679mg
Fiber: 7g PCF Ratio: 19-54-26 Exchange Approx.: 2 Starches, 1½ Vegetables, 1 Lean Meat, 1 Very-Lean Meat, 3 Fats

INGREDIENTS | SERVES 5

2 cups canned pinto beans, drained and rinsed
2 cups canned diced tomatoes
½ cup water
1 cup diced onion
2 teaspoons Cajun Blend seasoning (see Chapter 17)
8 ounces turkey kielbasa sausage, cut into 1" pieces
½ cup brown rice
1½ cups water

1. Combine the pinto beans, canned tomatoes, water, onion, Cajun seasoning, and kielbasa in a slow cooker. Set on low and cook for 4–6 hours.

2. In separate saucepan, bring the brown rice and 1½ cups water to boil. Reduce heat and simmer on low heat for 35–40 minutes.

3. Serve beans and sausage over rice.

Honey and Cider Glaze for Baked Chicken

NUTRITIONAL ANALYSIS (per serving, glaze only)

Calories: 10 Protein: 0g Carbohydrates: 2g Fat: 0g Saturated Fat: 0g Cholesterol: 0mg Sodium: 55mg
Fiber: 0g PCF Ratio: 9-90-1 Exchange Approx.: 1 Free Condiment

INGREDIENTS | SERVES 4

3 tablespoons cider or apple juice
½ teaspoon honey
1 teaspoon lemon juice
1 teaspoon Bragg's Liquid Aminos
½ teaspoon lemon zest

Spice Tea Chicken Marinade

Steep 4 orange or lemon spice tea bags in 2 cups boiling water for 4 minutes. Dissolve 1 teaspoon honey into the tea, pour it over 4 chicken pieces, and marinate for 30 minutes. Occasionally turn and baste any exposed portions of chicken. Pour the tea into the roasting pan to provide moisture—discard it after cooking.

1. Preheat the oven to 375°F.

2. Combine all the ingredients in a microwave-safe bowl. Microwave on high for 30 seconds. Stir until honey is dissolved.

3. To use glaze, arrange 4 boneless chicken pieces with skin removed on rack placed in roasting pan or broiling pan. Brush or spoon 1 teaspoon of glaze over the top of each piece. Baste halfway through cooking time, and again 5 minutes before chicken is done. Allow chicken to sit for 5 minutes before serving.

CHAPTER 11

Fish and Seafood Dishes

Fish Stock

NUTRITIONAL ANALYSIS (per serving)

Calories: 40   Protein: 5g   Carbohydrates: 0g   Fat: 2g   Saturated Fat: 1g   Cholesterol: 2mg   Sodium: Variable
Fiber: 0g   PCF Ratio: 55-0-45   Exchange Approx.: 1 Very-Lean Meat

INGREDIENTS | YIELDS 4 CUPS; SERVING SIZE 1 CUP

4 cups fish heads, bones, and trimmings (approx. 1 pound)
2 stalks celery and leaves, chopped
1 onion, chopped
1 carrot, peeled and chopped
1 bay leaf
4 sprigs fresh parsley
Sea salt and pepper, to taste (optional)

Tip

To make stock from shellfish, simply substitute shrimp, crab, or lobster shells for the fish heads and bones.

1. Use your own fish trimmings (saved in bag in the freezer) or ask the butcher at your local fish market or supermarket for fish trimmings. Wash the trimmings well.

2. In a stockpot, combine all the ingredients. Add enough water to cover everything by an inch or so. Bring to a boil over high heat, then reduce heat to low. Skim off foam that rises to top. Cover and simmer for 20 minutes.

3. Remove from heat and strain through a sieve, discarding all solids. Refrigerate or freeze.

Asian-Style Fish Cakes

NUTRITIONAL ANALYSIS (per serving)

Calories: 66 Protein: 11g Carbohydrates: 1g Fat: 2g Saturated Fat: 1g Cholesterol: 41mg Sodium: 112mg
Fiber: 0mg PCF Ratio: 69-8-23 Exchange Approx.: 1 Lean Meat, 1 Free Condiment

INGREDIENTS | SERVES 8

1-pound catfish fillet

2 green onions, minced

1 banana pepper, cored, seeded, and chopped

2 cloves garlic, minced

1 tablespoon grated or minced ginger

1 tablespoon Bragg's Liquid Aminos

1 tablespoon lemon juice

1 teaspoon lemon zest

Old Bay Seasoning, optional (see Chapter 17)

Tip

For crunchy fish cakes, coat each side in rice flour and then lightly spritz the tops of the patties with olive or peanut oil before baking as directed.

1. Preheat the oven to 375°F. Cut the fish into 1" pieces.

2. In a food processor, combine the fish, green onions, banana pepper, garlic, ginger, Bragg's Liquid Aminos, lemon juice, and lemon zest and process until chopped and mixed. (You do not want to purée this mixture; it should be a rough chop.) Add Old Bay Seasoning, if using, and stir to mix.

3. Form fish mixture into patties of about 2 tablespoons each; you should have 16 patties total.

4. Place patties on baking sheet treated with nonstick cooking spray and bake for 12–15 minutes, or until crisp. (Alternatively, you can fry these in a nonstick pan for about 4 minutes on each side.)

Salmon Patties

NUTRITIONAL ANALYSIS (per serving)

Calories: **168**   Protein: **17g**   Carbohydrates: **3g**   Fat: **9g**   Saturated Fat: **2g**   Cholesterol: **70mg**   Sodium: **92mg**
Fiber: **0g**   PCF Ratio: **42-8-50**   Exchange Approx.: **2 Lean Meats, ½ Fat, ½ Starch**

INGREDIENTS | SERVES 5

2 cups flaked cooked salmon (no salt added)

6 soda crackers, crushed

1 egg

½ cup skim milk

1 small onion, chopped

1 tablespoon fresh parsley, chopped

1 tablespoon unbleached all-purpose flour

1 tablespoon olive oil

Ener-G rice flour (optional)

1. Place the salmon in a bowl and flake with a fork.

2. Add the crushed crackers, egg, milk, onion, parsley, and all-purpose flour and mix well. Gently form 5 patties.

3. Heat oil in nonstick skillet over medium heat. (Optional: Lightly dust patties with some Ener-G rice flour for crispier patties.) Fry on both sides until browned, about 5 minutes per side.

Crab Cakes with Sesame Crust

NUTRITIONAL ANALYSIS (per serving)

Calories: 220   Protein: 20g   Carbohydrates: 8g   Fat: 12g   Saturated Fat: 2g   Cholesterol: 85mg   Sodium: 907mg
Fiber: 2g   PCF Ratio: 34-14-50   Exchange Approx.: 3 Very-Lean Meat, 2 Fats, ½ Starch

INGREDIENTS | SERVES 5

1 pound (16 ounces) lump crabmeat

1 egg

1 tablespoon minced fresh ginger

1 small scallion, finely chopped

1 tablespoon dry sherry

1 tablespoon freshly squeezed lemon juice

6 tablespoons real mayonnaise

Sea salt and freshly ground white pepper, to taste (optional)

Old Bay Seasoning to taste, optional (see Chapter 17)

¼ cup lightly toasted sesame seeds

1. Preheat the oven to 375°F.

2. In a large bowl, mix together the crab, egg, ginger, scallion, sherry, lemon juice, mayonnaise, and seasonings, if using. Form the mixture into 10 equal cakes.

3. Spread the sesame seeds over a sheet pan. Dip both sides of the cakes into the seeds to coat them.

4. Arrange cakes on a baking sheet treated with nonstick spray. Typical baking time is 8–10 minutes, depending on thickness of cakes.

Barley-Spinach-Fish Bake

NUTRITIONAL ANALYSIS (per serving)

Calories: 239   Protein: 26g   Carbohydrates: 15g   Fat: 8g   Saturated Fat: 1g   Cholesterol: 67mg   Sodium: 418mg
Fiber: 3g   PCF Ratio: 44-26-30   Exchange Approx.: 3 Lean Meats, ½ Starch, 1 Vegetable, 1½ Fats

INGREDIENTS | SERVES 4

½ tablespoon olive oil

¼ cup chopped scallions

1 clove garlic, minced

¼ teaspoon rosemary

¼ teaspoon marjoram

¼ teaspoon salt

1 cup cooked pearl barley

5 ounces (½ box) frozen chopped spinach, thawed and drained

¼ cup sundried tomatoes, chopped

4 (12-inch) squares of aluminum foil

4 (4-ounce) fish fillets

3 tablespoons white wine

Salt and fresh ground pepper, to taste

Cooking Barley

Pearl barley takes longer to cook than quick-cooking barley, so you will want to prepare it in advance. To prepare: Bring ½ cup pearl barley and 1 cup water to a boil. Reduce heat, cover, and simmer for 35–45 minutes, or until all water is absorbed. Pearl barley makes a good side dish on its own with the addition of spices or vegetables.

1. Preheat the oven to 400°F (or outdoor grill can be used).

2. Heat oil in a medium nonstick skillet. Add the scallions and sauté for 2 minutes.

3. Add the garlic, rosemary, marjoram, and salt and continue to cook for another 3 minutes, until scallions are tender.

4. Add the cooked barley, spinach, and sundried tomatoes, and mix well.

5. Place the aluminum foil squares on a work surface. Place a fish fillet in center of each square. Divide barley mixture equally on top of each fillet. Sprinkle with white wine, salt, and pepper.

6. Fold aluminum foil loosely to enclose filling. Place packets on baking sheet (or directly on grill if using outdoor grill) and bake for 15 minutes, or until fish is tender and flakes easily.

Grilled Salmon with Roasted Peppers

NUTRITIONAL ANALYSIS (per serving)

Calories: **269**   Protein: **24g**   Carbohydrates: **8g**   Fat: **16g**   Saturated Fat: **3g**   Cholesterol: **67mg**   Sodium: **321mg**
Fiber: **1g**   PCF Ratio: **36-11-53**   Exchange Approx.: **3½ Lean Meats, 1 Vegetable, 1 Fat**

INGREDIENTS | SERVES 4

4 (4-ounce) salmon steaks
1 tablespoon reduced-sodium soy sauce
1 tablespoon brown sugar
1 tablespoon olive oil
2 large red bell peppers
1 tablespoon balsamic vinegar
½ teaspoon dried thyme
¼ teaspoon fresh-ground pepper

Wasabi Marinade

Wasabi, also known as Japanese horseradish, can be purchased in raw form or as a powder or paste. It adds a hot, pungent flavor to fish and works especially well with salmon. To make a marinade for salmon or other fish, mix 1 teaspoon wasabi powder (or paste) with 2 tablespoons low-sodium soy sauce, ½ teaspoon grated ginger, and 1 teaspoon sesame oil. Coat fish with the marinade and grill.

1. Place the salmon in a shallow dish.

2. In a small bowl, mix together the soy sauce, brown sugar, and olive oil. Pour over the salmon and cover both sides with marinade. Set aside.

3. Prepare roasted red peppers following procedure discussed in the Roasted Red Pepper and Plum Sauce recipe in Chapter 16. Once peppers are roasted and peeled, cut into strips and sprinkle with balsamic vinegar, thyme, and pepper. Set aside.

4. Heat grill. Remove salmon from the marinade and grill it over medium heat for approximately 8 minutes on one side. Turn and grill on other side until salmon is cooked and tender, about 4–5 minutes longer. Remove from heat.

5. Top each salmon steak with marinated roasted red peppers.

Baked Bread Crumb–Crusted Fish with Lemon

NUTRITIONAL ANALYSIS (per serving, without salt)

Calories: **137**   Protein: **24g**   Carbohydrates: **5g**   Fat: **3g**   Saturated Fat: **1g**   Cholesterol: **36mg**   Sodium: **73mg**
Fiber: **2g**   PCF Ratio: **68-14-18**   Exchange Approx.: **2 Very-Lean Meats, ½ Starch, ½ Free Condiment**

INGREDIENTS | SERVES 6

2 large lemons
¼ cup dried bread crumbs
1½ pounds (24 ounces) halibut fillets
Sea or kosher salt and freshly ground white or black pepper, to taste (optional)

Lemon Infusion

Mildly flavored fish such as catfish, cod, halibut, orange roughy, rockfish, and snapper benefit from the distinctive flavor of lemon. Adding slices of lemon to the top of fish allows the flavor to infuse into the fish.

1. Preheat the oven to 375°F.

2. Wash 1 lemon and cut into thin slices. Grate 1 tablespoon of zest from the second lemon, then juice it.

3. Combine grated zest and bread crumbs in small bowl and stir to mix. Set aside.

4. Put lemon juice in shallow dish. Arrange lemon slices on the bottom of a baking dish treated with nonstick spray.

5. Dip fish pieces in the lemon juice and set on the lemon slices in the baking dish.

6. Sprinkle bread crumb mixture evenly over fish pieces along with salt and pepper, if using. Bake until crumbs are lightly browned and fish is just opaque, about 10–15 minutes. (Baking time will depend on thickness of fish.) Serve immediately, using lemon slices as garnish.

Baked Red Snapper Amandine

NUTRITIONAL ANALYSIS (per serving, without salt)

Calories: **178**   Protein: **24g**   Carbohydrates: **3g**   Fat: **7g**   Saturated Fat: **2g**   Cholesterol: **47mg**   Sodium: **73mg**
Fiber: **1g**   PCF Ratio: **56-7-37**   Exchange Approx.: **3 Lean Meats**

INGREDIENTS | SERVES 4

1 pound (16 ounces) red snapper fillets

Sea or kosher salt and freshly ground white or black pepper, to taste (optional)

4 teaspoons all-purpose flour

2 teaspoons olive oil

2 tablespoons ground raw almonds

2 teaspoons unsalted butter

1 tablespoon lemon juice

1. Preheat the oven to 375°F.

2. Rinse red snapper fillets and dry between layers of paper towels. Season with salt and pepper, if using. Sprinkle with flour, front and back.

3. In an ovenproof nonstick skillet, sauté the fillets in olive oil until nicely browned on both sides, about 5 minutes per side.

4. Combine ground almonds and butter in microwave-safe dish. Microwave on high for 30 seconds, or until butter is melted. Stir to combine.

5. Pour almond-butter mixture and lemon juice over fillets and bake for 3–5 minutes, or until almonds are nicely browned.

A-Taste-of-Italy Baked Fish

NUTRITIONAL ANALYSIS (per serving)

Calories: **128**   Protein: **22g**   Carbohydrates: **7g**   Fat: **1g**   Saturated Fat: **0g**   Cholesterol: **50mg**   Sodium: **312mg**
Fiber: **1g**   PCF Ratio: **68-23-9**   Exchange Approx.: **2½ Very-Lean Meats, 1½ Vegetables**

INGREDIENTS | SERVES 4

1 pound (16 ounces) cod fillets
1 (14½-ounce) can stewed tomatoes
¼ teaspoon dried minced onion
½ teaspoon dried minced garlic
¼ teaspoon dried basil
¼ teaspoon dried parsley
⅛ teaspoon dried oregano
⅛ teaspoon sugar
1 tablespoon grated Parmesan cheese

1. Preheat the oven to 375°F.

2. Rinse the cod with cold water and pat dry with paper towels.

3. In a 2–3-quart baking pan or casserole treated with nonstick cooking spray, combine all the ingredients except fish, and mix.

4. Arrange fillets over mixture, folding thin tail ends under; spoon mixture over fillets. For fillets about 1" thick, bake uncovered for 20–25 minutes, or until fish is opaque and flaky.

Crunchy "Fried" Catfish Fillets

NUTRITIONAL ANALYSIS (per serving, without salt)

Calories: 244 Protein: 21g Carbohydrates: 18g Fat: 9g Saturated Fat: 2g Cholesterol: 53mg Sodium: 248mg
Fiber: 1g PCF Ratio: 35-30-35 Exchange Approx.: 3 Lean Meats, 1 Starch

INGREDIENTS | SERVES 4

4 (3-ounce) catfish fillets

1 egg white (from a large egg), room temperature

¼ cup bread crumbs

¼ cup enriched white cornmeal

1 teaspoon grated lemon zest

½ teaspoon crushed dried basil

¼ cup all-purpose flour

⅛ teaspoon kosher or sea salt (optional)

¼ teaspoon lemon pepper

Zesty Crunch

Grated lemon or lime zest is a great way to give added citrus flavor to a crunchy bread-crumb topping for fish.

1. Preheat the oven to 450°F. Treat a shallow baking pan with nonstick spray.

2. Rinse catfish and dry between layers of paper towels.

3. In shallow dish, beat the egg white until frothy.

4. In another dish, combine the bread crumbs, cornmeal, lemon zest, and basil.

5. In a third dish, combine the flour, salt (if using), and lemon pepper.

6. Dip the fish into flour mixture to coat 1 side of each fillet. Shake off any excess flour mixture, then dip flour-covered side of fillet into egg white. Next, coat covered side of fillet with bread-crumb mixture.

7. Arrange prepared fillets side by side, coated-sides up, on prepared baking pan. Tuck in any thin edges. Bake for 6–12 minutes, or until fish flakes easily with a fork.

Jon's Fish Tacos

NUTRITIONAL ANALYSIS (per serving)

Calories: 383   Protein: 29g   Carbohydrates: 40g   Fat: 12g   Saturated Fat: 2g   Cholesterol: 60mg   Sodium: 400mg
Fiber: 4g   PCF Ratio: 30-42-28   Exchange Approx.: 3½ Very-Lean Meats, 2 Starches, 1 Vegetable, 1 Fat

INGREDIENTS | SERVES 4

¼ cup light mayonnaise
½ cup plain nonfat yogurt
¼ cup chopped onion
2 tablespoons minced jalapeño pepper
2 teaspoons minced cilantro
2 cups shredded cabbage
¼ cup lime juice
1 clove garlic, minced
1 tablespoon canola oil
1 pound tilapia fillets
Aluminum foil
Nonstick cooking spray
4 whole-wheat tortillas, 6" diameter
1 cup chopped tomato
Fresh ground pepper, to taste

1. In medium bowl, whisk together the mayonnaise, yogurt, onion, jalapeño, and cilantro. Stir in shredded cabbage. Chill.

2. In a separate bowl, combine the lime juice, garlic, and canola oil to make a marinade for the fish. Pour over the fish; cover and refrigerate for at least 1 hour.

3. Place fish on aluminum-lined grill (spray aluminum with cooking spray) and cook for 6–7 minutes on each side, until fish is tender and beginning to flake.

4. While the fish is cooking, loosely wrap whole-wheat tortillas in large piece of aluminum foil and place on grill to heat.

5. To assemble tacos, cut the fish into strips and divide into 4 portions. Place strips in center of each heated tortilla. Top with coleslaw mixture and chopped tomatoes. Add fresh ground pepper, if desired.

Sweet Onion–Baked Yellowtail Snapper

NUTRITIONAL ANALYSIS (per serving, no salt)

Calories: **189**   Protein: **25g**   Carbohydrates: **13g**   Fat: **4g**   Saturated Fat: **1g**   Cholesterol: **42mg**   Sodium: **77mg**
Fiber: **1g**   PCF Ratio: **53-28-19**   Exchange Approx.: **1 Lean Meat, 2 Very-Lean Meats, 1 Vegetable, ½ Starch**

INGREDIENTS | SERVES 4

2 cups sliced Vidalia onions

1 tablespoon balsamic vinegar

2 teaspoons brown sugar

4 teaspoons olive oil

1 pound (16 ounces) skinless yellowtail snapper fillets

Sea salt and freshly ground white or black pepper, to taste (optional)

1. In covered microwave-safe dish, microwave onion on high for 5 minutes, or until transparent. Carefully remove cover and stir in vinegar and brown sugar. Cover and allow to sit for several minutes so onion absorbs flavors.

2. Heat a nonstick pan on medium-high and add the olive oil. Transfer steamed onion mixture to pan and sauté until browned but not crisp. (Be careful, as onions will burn easily because of brown sugar; if onion browns too quickly, lower heat and add a few tablespoons of water.) Cook until all liquid has evaporated from pan, stirring often, approximately 2 minutes. Onions should have a shiny and dark caramelized color. (This can be prepared 2–3 days in advance; store tightly covered in refrigerator.)

3. Preheat the oven to 375°F.

4. Rinse the snapper in cold water and dry between paper towels. Arrange on baking sheet treated with nonstick spray.

5. Spoon caramelized onions over tops of fillets, pressing to form a light crust over top of fish. Bake for 12–15 minutes, or until fish flakes easily with a fork. Serve immediately divided on 4 plates with fish placed on top. Add sea salt and freshly ground white or black pepper, to taste (optional)

Stir-Fried Ginger Scallops with Vegetables

NUTRITIONAL ANALYSIS (per serving)

Calories: 145   Protein: 22g   Carbohydrates: 8g   Fat: 3g   Saturated Fat: 1g   Cholesterol: 37mg   Sodium: 373mg
Fiber: 2g   PCF Ratio: 61-23-16   Exchange Approx.: 3 Very-Lean Meats, ½ Vegetable

INGREDIENTS | SERVES 4

1 pound (16 ounces) scallops

1 teaspoon peanut or sesame oil

1 tablespoon chopped fresh ginger

2 cloves garlic, minced

4 scallions, thinly sliced (optional)

1 teaspoon rice wine vinegar

2 teaspoons Bragg's Liquid Aminos

½ cup low-fat reduced-sodium chicken broth

2 cups broccoli florets

1 teaspoon cornstarch

¼ teaspoon toasted sesame oil

1. Rinse scallops and pat dry between layers of paper towels. Set aside.

2. Add peanut oil to heated nonstick deep skillet or wok. Sauté ginger, garlic, and scallions, if using, for 1–2 minutes. Add vinegar, Liquid Aminos, and broth, and bring to a boil. Remove from heat.

3. Place broccoli in a large, covered microwave-safe dish. Pour chicken broth mixture over top. Microwave on high for 3–5 minutes, depending on preference. (Keep in mind that vegetables will continue to steam for a minute or so if cover remains on dish.)

4. Heat skillet or wok over medium-high temperature. Add scallops and sauté for 1 minute on each side. (Do scallops in batches if necessary; be careful not to overcook.) Remove scallops from pan when done and set aside.

5. Drain (but do not discard) liquid from broccoli. Return liquid to bowl and transfer broccoli to heated skillet or wok. Stir-fry vegetables to bring up to serving temperature.

6. Meanwhile, in small cup or bowl, add ¼ cup water to cornstarch to make a slurry or roux. Whisk slurry into reserved broccoli liquid and microwave on high for 1 minute.

7. Add toasted sesame oil and whisk again.

8. Pour broth mixture over broccoli and toss to mix.

9. Add scallops back to broccoli mixture and stir-fry over medium heat to return scallops to serving temperature. Serve over rice or pasta; adjust Exchange Approximations accordingly.

Scallops and Shrimp with White Bean Sauce

NUTRITIONAL ANALYSIS (per serving)

Calories: 231   Protein: 27g   Carbohydrates: 18g   Fat: 4g   Saturated Fat: 1g   Cholesterol: 105mg   Sodium: 217mg
Fiber: 7g   PCF Ratio: 49-34-17   Exchange Approx.: 3 Very-Lean Meats, ½ Fat, 1 Starch, ½ Vegetable

INGREDIENTS | SERVES 4

½ cup finely chopped onion, steamed

2 cloves garlic, minced

2 teaspoons olive oil, divided

¼ cup dry white wine

¼ cup tightly packed fresh parsley leaves

¼ cup tightly packed fresh basil leaves

1⅓ cups canned cannellini (white) beans, drained and rinsed

¼ cup low-fat, reduced-sodium chicken broth

½ pound (8 ounces) shrimp, shelled and deveined

½ pound (8 ounces) scallops

1. In nonstick saucepan over moderately low heat, sauté the onion and garlic in 1 teaspoon of oil for about 5 minutes until onion is soft.

2. Add the wine and simmer until wine is reduced by half.

3. Add parsley, basil, ⅓ cup of beans, and chicken broth. Simmer, stirring constantly, for 1 minute.

4. Transfer bean mixture to blender or food processor and purée. Pour purée back into saucepan and add remaining beans; simmer for 2 minutes.

5. In nonstick skillet over moderately high heat, heat remaining 1 teaspoon of oil until it is hot but not smoking. Sauté shrimp for 2 minutes on each side, or until cooked through. Using slotted spoon, transfer shrimp to plate; cover to keep warm.

6. Add scallops to skillet and sauté for 1 minute on each side, or until cooked through.

7. To serve, divide bean sauce between 4 shallow bowls and arrange shellfish over top.

Pasta and Smoked Trout with Lemon Pesto

NUTRITIONAL ANALYSIS (per serving)

Calories: **209** Protein: **10g** Carbohydrates: **23g** Fat: **8g** Saturated Fat: **1g** Cholesterol: **4mg** Sodium: **151mg**
Fiber: **1g** PCF Ratio: **20-45-36** Exchange Approx.: **1 Fat, 1½ Lean Meats, 1 Carbohydrate/Starch**

INGREDIENTS | SERVES 4

2 cloves garlic

2 cups fresh basil leaves, tightly packed

⅛ cup pine nuts, toasted

2 teaspoons fresh lemon juice

2 teaspoons water

4 teaspoons extra-virgin olive oil

4 tablespoons grated Parmesan cheese, divided

1⅓ cups uncooked linguini or other pasta (to yield 2 cups cooked pasta)

2 ounces whole boneless smoked trout

Freshly ground black pepper, to taste

1. Put the garlic in food processor and pulse until finely chopped.

2. Add the basil, pine nuts, lemon juice, and water and process until just puréed. (Note: You can substitute fresh parsley for basil; supplement flavor by adding some dried basil, too, if you do.)

3. Add olive oil and 3 tablespoons of Parmesan cheese. Pulse until pesto is smooth, occasionally scraping down side of bowl, if necessary. Set aside.

4. Cook pasta according to package directions. While it is cooking, flake trout.

5. When pasta is cooked, pulse pesto to ensure it has remained blended. Toss pesto and trout with pasta. Sprinkle remaining Parmesan and some pepper on top of each serving. (Although this recipe uses heart-healthy extra-virgin olive oil, it is a little higher in fat, but still low in calories. Consult your dietitian if you have any question whether you should include this recipe in your meal plans.)

Grilled Haddock with Peach-Mango Salsa

NUTRITIONAL ANALYSIS (per serving, including ½ cup peach-mango salsa)

Calories: 204 Protein: 22g Carbohydrates: 11g Fat: 8g Saturated Fat: 1g Cholesterol: 65mg Sodium: 467mg
Fiber: 2g PCF Ratio: 43-22-35 Exchange Approx.: 3 Very-Lean Meats, 1 Fat, ½ Fruit

INGREDIENTS | SERVES 4

2 tablespoons olive oil
2 tablespoons lime juice
¼ teaspoon salt
¼ teaspoon ground pepper
1 pound haddock fillets
Fresh Peach-Mango Salsa (see Chapter 16)

1. In a shallow dish, combine the olive oil, lime juice, salt, and pepper.

2. Add haddock to the dish. Turn and coat fish with marinade.

3. Heat gas grill or broiler. Spray large piece of aluminum foil with nonstick cooking spray. Place fillets on foil and cook for 7–8 minutes on each side, or until fish is tender when pierced with a fork.

4. Top each piece of fish with ½ cup Fresh Peach-Mango Salsa.

Sesame Shrimp and Asparagus

NUTRITIONAL ANALYSIS (per serving)

Calories: 257   Protein: 28g   Carbohydrates: 23g   Fat: 6g   Saturated Fat: 1g   Cholesterol: 172mg   Sodium: 173mg
Fiber: 3g   PCF Ratio: 44-35-21   Exchange Approx.: 3 Very-Lean Meats, ½ Vegetable, 1 Starch

INGREDIENTS | SERVES 4

2 teaspoons canola oil

2 cloves garlic, chopped

1 tablespoon grated fresh gingerroot

1 pound medium shrimp

2 tablespoons dry white wine

½ pound asparagus, cut diagonally into 1" pieces

2 cups whole-grain pasta, cooked

½ teaspoon sesame seeds

¼ cup scallions, thinly sliced

1 teaspoon sesame oil

1. Heat canola oil in a wok or large nonstick skillet. Stir-fry the garlic, gingerroot, and shrimp over high heat until shrimp begins to turn pink, about 2 minutes.

2. Add white wine and asparagus. Stir-fry for an additional 3–5 minutes.

3. Add pasta, sesame seeds, scallions, and sesame oil. Toss lightly and serve.

Spicy "Fried" Fish Fillet

NUTRITIONAL ANALYSIS (per serving)

Calories: 230   Protein: 24g   Carbohydrates: 9g   Fat: 10g   Saturated Fat: 2g   Cholesterol: 116mg   Sodium: 412mg
Fiber: 1g   PCF Ratio: 44-17-39   Exchange Approx.: 3 Very-Lean Meats, 2 Fats, ½ Starch

INGREDIENTS | SERVES 4

⅓ cup cornmeal
½ teaspoon salt
1 teaspoon chipotle seasoning
1 egg
2 tablespoons 1% milk
16 ounces flounder, cut into 4 pieces
2 tablespoons olive oil

1. Combine cornmeal, salt, and chipotle seasoning in shallow dish.

2. In another shallow dish, beat the egg and milk together.

3. Dip the fish in the egg mixture and then coat each fillet with the cornmeal mixture.

4. Heat olive oil in nonstick skillet. Brown fillets until golden and crispy, about 6–7 minutes each side.

Fresh Tomato and Clam Sauce with Whole-Grain Linguini

NUTRITIONAL ANALYSIS (per serving)

Calories: 361   Protein: 13g   Carbohydrates: 60g   Fat: 8g   Saturated Fat: 1g   Cholesterol: 7mg   Sodium: 356mg
Fiber: 8g   PCF Ratio: 14-66-20   Exchange Approx.: 2½ Starches, 1½ Very-Lean Meats, 3 Vegetables, 1½ Fats

INGREDIENTS | SERVES 4

3 dozen (36) littleneck clams

½ cup cornmeal

2 tablespoons olive oil

5 cloves garlic, chopped

½ cup chopped red bell pepper

4 cups peeled and chopped fresh tomatoes

3 tablespoons chopped fresh parsley

1 tablespoon chopped fresh basil

¼ teaspoon salt

¼ teaspoon red pepper flakes

½ teaspoon dried oregano

½ cup dry white wine

8 ounces whole-grain linguini

Tip

This recipe works well with canned clams if you are unable to get fresh. Canned clams are quite high in sodium, which will need to be taken into consideration. If using canned clams, you will need 1 (8-ounce) can of minced clams and 1 (10-ounce) can of whole clams. Reserve the clam juice and add to the sauce.

1. Before preparing this dish (preferably several hours or more), place clams in bowl of cold water with cornmeal added. Keep refrigerated. (This will help purge clams of any sand or other debris.) When ready to cook, rinse and scrub clams.

2. Heat the olive oil, garlic, and red pepper in a deep skillet. Add chopped tomatoes, parsley, basil, salt, red pepper flakes, and oregano, and bring to quick boil. Reduce the heat and simmer for 15–20 minutes.

3. Stir in white wine. Add clams on top of tomato sauce. Cover and steam until clams open, approximately 3–4 minutes.

4. Meanwhile, boil water and cook pasta to al dente.

5. Serve tomato sauce and clams over pasta.

CHAPTER 12

Casseroles and Stews

Condensed Cream of Mushroom Soup

NUTRITIONAL ANALYSIS (per recipe)

Calories: 92   Protein: 3g   Carbohydrates: 21g   Fat: 1g   Saturated Fat: 0g   Cholesterol: 0mg   Sodium: 13mg
Fiber: 3g   PCF Ratio: 12-84-4   Exchange Approx.: Will depend on serving size and preparation method

INGREDIENTS	YIELDS EQUIVALENT OF 1 (10¾ OUNCE) CAN

¾ cup finely chopped fresh mushrooms

½ cup water

⅛ cup Ener-G potato flour

Optional ingredients:

1 teaspoon chopped onion

1 tablespoon chopped celery

½ cup water

⅛ cup Ener-G potato flour

Potato Flour Substitute?

Instant mashed potatoes can replace potato flour; however, the amount needed will vary according to the brand of potatoes. Also, you'll need to consider other factors such as added fats and hydrogenated oils.

1. In a microwave-safe covered container, microwave mushrooms (and onion and celery, if using) for 2 minutes, or until tender. (About ¾ cup chopped mushrooms will yield ½ cup steamed ones.) Reserve any resulting liquid; add enough water to equal 1 cup.

2. Place all the ingredients in a blender and process. The thickness of soup concentrate will vary according to how much moisture remains in mushrooms. If necessary, add 1–2 tablespoons of water to achieve a paste. (Low-sodium canned mushrooms work in this recipe, but the Nutritional Analysis assumes fresh mushrooms are used. Adjust sodium content accordingly.)

Condensed Cream of Chicken Soup

NUTRITIONAL ANALYSIS (per recipe)

Calories: **158**   Protein: **4g**   Carbohydrates: **35g**   Fat: **1g**   Saturated Fat: **0g**   Cholesterol: **1mg**   Sodium: **162mg**
Fiber: **1g**   PCF Ratio: **9-88-3**   Exchange Approx.: **Will depend on serving size and preparation method**

INGREDIENTS	YIELDS EQUIVALENT OF 1 (10¾ OUNCE) CAN

1 cup water

¾ teaspoon Minor's Low-Sodium Chicken Base

¼ cup Ener-G potato flour

Place all the ingredients in blender and process until well blended.

Condensed Cream of Chicken Soup with Regular Chicken Broth

For the equivalent of 1 (10¾ ounce) can of condensed chicken soup, blend 1 cup reduced-fat canned chicken broth with ¼ cup Ener-G potato flour. It will last, refrigerated, for 3 days. Nutritional Analysis: Calories: 181.20; Protein: 7.61g; Carbohydrates: 34.14g; Fat: 1.50g; Saturated Fat: 0.42g; Cholesterol: 0.00mg; Sodium: 785.20mg; Fiber: 2.36g; PCF Ratio: 17-76-7; Exchange Approx.: will depend on serving size and preparation method.

Condensed Cream of Celery Soup

NUTRITIONAL ANALYSIS (per recipe)

Calories: 85   Protein: 2g   Carbohydrates: 20g   Fat: 0g   Saturated Fat: 0g   Cholesterol: 0mg   Sodium: 79mg
Fiber: 2g   PCF Ratio: 9-89-2   Exchange Approx.: Will depend on serving size and preparation method

INGREDIENTS	YIELDS EQUIVALENT OF 1 (10¾ OUNCE) CAN

½ cup steamed chopped celery
½ cup water
⅛ cup Ener-G potato flour

1. In a microwave-safe, covered container, microwave the celery for 2 minutes, or until tender. Do not drain any resulting liquid. If necessary, add enough water to bring celery and liquid to 1 cup total.

2. Place all the ingredients, including the rest of the 1 cup water, in blender and process. Use immediately, or store in a covered container in refrigerator for use within 3 days. Thickness of concentrate will depend on how much moisture remains in celery. Add 1–2 tablespoons of water, if necessary, to achieve a paste.

Condensed Cream of Potato Soup

NUTRITIONAL ANALYSIS (per recipe)

Calories: **103** Protein: **2g** Carbohydrates: **24g** Fat: **0g** Saturated Fat: **0g** Cholesterol: **0mg** Sodium: **9mg**
Fiber: **2g** PCF Ratio: **8-91-1** Exchange Approx.: **Will depend on serving size and preparation method**

INGREDIENTS	YIELDS EQUIVALENT OF 1 (10¾ OUNCE) CAN

½ cup peeled, diced potatoes
½ cup water
1 tablespoon Ener-G potato flour

Tip
The Nutritional Analysis for this recipe assumes you'll use the entire tablespoon of Ener-G potato flour; however, the amount needed will depend on the amount of starch in the potatoes you use. For example, new potatoes will require more Ener-G potato flour than larger, Idaho-style potatoes.

1. Place potatoes and water in a covered microwave-safe bowl. Microwave on high for 4–5 minutes, until potatoes are fork-tender.

2. Pour potatoes and water in a blender, being careful of steam. Remove vent from blender lid and process until smooth.

3. Add Ener-G flour 1 teaspoon at a time while blender is running.

Condensed Tomato Soup

NUTRITIONAL ANALYSIS (per recipe)

Calories: **136**   Protein: **4g**   Carbohydrates: **31g**   Fat: **1g**   Saturated Fat: **0g**   Cholesterol: **0mg**   Sodium: **352mg**
Fiber: **4g**   PCF Ratio: **11-83-6**   Exchange Approx.: **Will depend on serving size and preparation method**

INGREDIENTS	YIELDS EQUIVALENT OF 1 (10¾ OUNCE) CAN

1 cup peeled chopped tomato, with juice

Additional tomato juices (if necessary)

¼ teaspoon baking soda

⅛ cup Ener-G potato flour

Direct Preparation

If you'll be making the soup immediately after you prepare the condensed soup recipe, you can simply add your choice of the additional 1 cup of liquid (such as skim milk, soy milk, or water) to the blender and use that method to mix the milk and soup concentrate together. Pour the combined mixture into your pan or microwave-safe dish.

1. Place tomato in microwave-safe bowl and microwave on high for 2–3 minutes, until tomato is cooked. Add additional tomato juices if necessary to bring mixture back up to 1 cup.

2. Add baking soda and stir vigorously until bubbling stops.

3. Pour cooked tomato mixture into blender.

4. Add potato flour, 1 tablespoon at a time, processing until well blended.

Condensed Cheese Soup

NUTRITIONAL ANALYSIS (per recipe)

Calories: 315 Protein: 20g Carbohydrates: 18g Fat: 18g Saturated Fat: 11g Cholesterol: 56mg Sodium: 384mg
Fiber: 1g PCF Ratio: 26-23-51 Exchange Approx.: Will depend on serving size and preparation method

INGREDIENTS	YIELDS EQUIVALENT OF 1 (10¾ OUNCE) CAN

½ cup water

⅛ cup Ener-G potato flour

¼ cup nonfat cottage cheese

2 ounces American, Cheddar, or Colby cheese, shredded (to yield ½ cup)

1. Place the water, potato flour, and cottage cheese in blender and process until well blended.

2. Stir in the shredded cheese. Cheese will melt as casserole is baked, prepared in microwave, or cooked on stovetop, according to recipe instructions.

Be Aware of Your Exchanges

When using any soup preparation method, you'll need to add the appropriate Exchange Approximations for each serving amount (usually ¼ of the total) of whatever condensed soup you make. For example, broth-based soups like chicken and cream of mushroom or celery would be a Free Exchange; cream of potato soup would add 1 Carbohydrate/Starch.

Soup Preparation Method

NUTRITIONAL ANALYSIS (per serving)

Additional Calories: 21   Protein: 2g   Carbohydrates: 3g   Fat: 0g   Saturated Fat: 0g   Cholesterol: 1mg   Sodium: 32mg
Fiber: 0g   PCF Ratio: 39-56-5   Exchange Approx.: 1 Low-Fat Milk for entire pot of soup; divide accordingly per serving

INGREDIENTS | SERVES 4

Any previous condensed soup recipe
1 cup skim milk

1. To use any of the homemade condensed soup recipes as soup, add 1 cup of skim milk (or soy milk or water) to a pan. Stir using a spoon or whisk to blend.

2. Cook over medium heat for 10 minutes until mixture begins to simmer. Season according to taste.

Traditional Stovetop Tuna-Noodle Casserole

NUTRITIONAL ANALYSIS (per serving, noodles cooked without salt)

Calories: 245 Protein: 20g Carbohydrates: 33g Fat: 4g Saturated Fat: 2g Cholesterol: 46mg Sodium: 241mg
Fiber: 4g PCF Ratio: 32-53-15 Exchange Approx.: 1½ Starches, 1 Vegetable, 1 Medium-Fat Meat

INGREDIENTS | SERVES 4

1⅓ cups egg noodles (yields 2 cups when cooked)

1 recipe Condensed Cream of Mushroom Soup (see recipe in this chapter)

1 teaspoon steamed chopped onion

1 tablespoon steamed chopped celery

½ cup skim milk

1 ounce American, Cheddar, or Colby cheese, shredded (to yield ¼ cup)

1 cup frozen mixed peas and carrots

1 cup steamed sliced fresh mushrooms

1 can water-packed tuna, drained

1. Cook egg noodles according to package directions. Drain and return to pan.

2. Add all the remaining ingredients to pan and stir to blend. Cook over medium heat, stirring occasionally, until cheese is melted.

Extra-Rich Stovetop Tuna-Noodle Casserole

Add 1 medium egg (beaten) and 1 tablespoon mayonnaise to give the casserole the taste of rich, homemade egg noodles while still maintaining a good fat ratio. It's still less than 300 calories per serving, too! Nutritional Analysis: Calories: 275; Protein: 21g; Carbohydrates: 34g; Fat: 7g; Saturated Fat: 2g; Cholesterol: 94mg; Sodium: 281mg; Fiber: 4g; PCF Ratio: 30-48-21; Exchange Approx.: 1½ Breads, 1 Vegetable, 1 Meat, 1 Medium-Fat Meat.

Chicken and Mushroom Rice Casserole

NUTRITIONAL ANALYSIS (per serving)

Calories: 165 Protein: 9g Carbohydrates: 30g Fat: 1g Saturated Fat: 0g Cholesterol: 15mg Sodium: 41mg
Fiber: 3g PCF Ratio: 23-71-6 Exchange Approx.: 1 Very-Lean Meat, 1 Starch, 1 Vegetable

INGREDIENTS | SERVES 8

1 recipe Condensed Cream of Chicken Soup (see recipe in this chapter)

1 cup diced chicken breast

1 large onion, chopped

½ cup chopped celery

1 cup uncooked rice (not instant rice)

Freshly ground black pepper, to taste (optional)

1 teaspoon dried Herbes de Provence Blend (see Chapter 17), optional

2 cups boiling water

2½ cups chopped broccoli florets

1 cup sliced fresh mushrooms

1. Preheat oven to 350°F.

2. In a 4-quart casserole dish (large enough to prevent boilovers in oven) treated with nonstick spray, combine the condensed soup, chicken breast, onion, celery, rice, and seasonings and mix well.

3. Pour boiling water over top and bake, covered, for 30 minutes.

4. Stir casserole. Add broccoli and mushrooms. Replace cover and return to oven to bake for an additional 20–30 minutes, or until celery is tender and rice has absorbed all liquid.

Ham and Artichoke Hearts Scalloped Potatoes

NUTRITIONAL ANALYSIS (per serving, without salt)

Calories: **269** Protein: **21g** Carbohydrates: **31g** Fat: **8g** Saturated Fat: **4g** Cholesterol: **28mg** Sodium: **762mg**
Fiber: **6g** PCF Ratio: **31-44-25** Exchange Approx.: **1½ Lean Meats, ½ High-Fat Meat, 1½ Vegetables, 1 Starch**

INGREDIENTS | SERVES 4

2 cups frozen artichoke hearts

1 cup chopped onion

4 small potatoes, thinly sliced

Sea salt and freshly ground black pepper, to taste (optional)

1 tablespoon lemon juice

1 tablespoon dry white wine

1 cup Mock Cream (see Chapter 16)

½ cup nonfat cottage cheese

1 teaspoon dried parsley

1 teaspoon garlic powder

⅛ cup freshly grated Parmesan cheese

¼ pound (4 ounces) lean ham, cubed

2 ounces Cheddar cheese, grated (to yield ½ cup)

Simple Substitutions

Artichoke hearts can be expensive. You can substitute cabbage, broccoli, or cauliflower (or a mixture of all 3) for the artichokes.

1. Preheat the oven to 300°F.

2. Thaw the artichoke hearts and pat dry with a paper towel.

3. In a deep casserole dish treated with nonstick spray, layer artichokes, onion, and potatoes and lightly sprinkle salt and pepper over top (if using).

4. In a food processor or blender, combine the lemon juice, wine, mock cream, cottage cheese, parsley, garlic powder, and Parmesan cheese. Process until smooth.

5. Pour cheese sauce over layered vegetables and top with ham. Cover casserole dish (with a lid or foil) and bake for 35–40 minutes, or until potatoes are cooked through.

6. Remove cover and top with Cheddar cheese. Return to oven for another 10 minutes, or until cheese is melted and bubbly. Let rest for 10 minutes before cutting.

Hearty Beef Stew (Fast and Slow Methods)

NUTRITIONAL ANALYSIS (per serving)

Calories: 326   Protein: 26g   Carbohydrates: 32g   Fat: 10g   Saturated Fat: 3g   Cholesterol: 88mg   Sodium: 335mg
Fiber: 4g   PCF Ratio: 32-39-28   Exchange Approx.: 3 Lean Meats, 1 Starch, 3 Vegetables

INGREDIENTS | SERVES 4

1 tablespoon olive oil

12 ounces beef round, cut into 1" cubes

1 cup chopped onion

2 cups potatoes, cut into 1" pieces

½ cup carrots, cut into 1" pieces

1 cup green beans

½ cup turnip, peeled and cut into 1" pieces

1 tablespoon parsley

¼ teaspoon Tabasco

1 cup low-sodium V8 juice

¼ teaspoon salt

1 tablespoon all-purpose flour

¼ cup water

1. Heat olive oil in a pressure cooker and brown meat.

2. Add the onions, potatoes, carrots, green beans, turnip, parsley, Tabasco, V8 juice, and salt.

3. Close cover securely. Place pressure regulator on vent pipe and cook for 10–12 minutes with pressure regulator rocking slowly. (Or follow manufacturer instructions for your pressure cooker.) Cool down pressure cooker at once (nonelectric pressure cookers).

4. If desired, make paste of 1 tablespoon flour and ¼ cup water and stir into the stew to thicken. Heat and stir liquid until thickened.

Slow-Cook Method for Beef Stew

If you don't have a pressure cooker, you can make this stew in a slow cooker. First, heat olive oil in a skillet. Dredge meat in 1–2 tablespoons flour; add to skillet and brown. Transfer to slow cooker; add onions, V8, potatoes, carrots, green beans, turnip, salt, parsley, and Tabasco. Cook on low-medium for 4–6 hours.

Main Dish Pork and Beans

NUTRITIONAL ANALYSIS (per serving)

Calories: **153** Protein: **11g** Carbohydrates: **24g** Fat: **2g** Saturated Fat: **1g** Cholesterol: **18mg** Sodium: **146mg**
Fiber: **5g** PCF Ratio: **29-61-10** Exchange Approx.: **2 Lean Meats, ½ Fruit/Misc. Carbohydrate**

INGREDIENTS | SERVES 4

1⅓ cups cooked pinto beans

2 tablespoons ketchup

¼ teaspoon Dijon mustard

¼ teaspoon dry mustard

1 teaspoon cider vinegar

4 tablespoons diced red onion

1 tablespoon 100% maple syrup

1 teaspoon brown sugar

¼ pound (4 ounces) slow-cooked shredded pork

⅛ cup (2 tablespoons) apple juice or cider

1. Preheat the oven to 350°F.

2. In casserole dish treated with nonstick spray, combine the beans, ketchup, Dijon mustard, dry mustard, vinegar, onion, syrup, and brown sugar.

3. Layer meat over top of bean mixture.

4. Pour apple juice or cider over pork. Bake for 20–30 minutes, or until mixture is well heated and bubbling. Stir well before serving.

Easy Oven Beef Burgundy

NUTRITIONAL ANALYSIS (per serving)

Calories: **266**   Protein: **34g**   Carbohydrates: **12g**   Fat: **6g**   Saturated Fat: **2g**   Cholesterol: **82mg**   Sodium: **388mg**
Fiber: **2g**   PCF Ratio: **56-20-23**   Exchange Approx.: **4 Lean Meats, 2 Vegetables, 1 Fat**

INGREDIENTS | SERVES 4

1 pound beef round, cubed
2 tablespoons all-purpose flour
1 cup sliced carrots
1 cup chopped onions
1 cup sliced celery
1 clove garlic, finely chopped
¼ teaspoon pepper
¼ teaspoon marjoram
¼ teaspoon thyme
½ teaspoon salt
2 tablespoons balsamic vinegar
½ cup dry red wine
½ cup water
1 cup sliced fresh mushrooms

1. Preheat the oven to 325°F.

2. Dredge meat cubes in flour. Place cubes in a 3-quart covered baking dish or Dutch oven.

3. Add carrots, onions, celery, garlic, pepper, marjoram, thyme, salt, and vinegar and stir to combine.

4. Pour red wine and water over mixture. Cover and bake for 1 hour.

5. Remove from oven and mix in the mushrooms.

6. Return to oven for 1 hour, or until beef cubes are tender.

Microwave Shrimp Casserole

NUTRITIONAL ANALYSIS (per serving)

Calories: 196 Protein: 18g Carbohydrates: 27g Fat: 2g Saturated Fat: 1g Cholesterol: 131mg Sodium: 290mg
Fiber: 2g PCF Ratio: 35-56-9 Exchange Approx.: 1 Starch, 1 Vegetable, 1 Medium-Fat Meat

INGREDIENTS | SERVES 4

1⅓ cups uncooked egg noodles

1 cup chopped green onion

1 cup chopped green pepper

1 cup sliced mushrooms

1 recipe Condensed Cream of Celery Soup (see recipe in this chapter)

1 teaspoon Worcestershire sauce (see recipe for Homemade Worcestershire in Chapter 16)

4 drops Tabasco (optional)

¼ cup diced canned pimientos

½ cup pitted, chopped ripe olives

½ cup skimmed milk

½ pound (8 ounces) cooked, deveined, shelled shrimp

1. Cook egg noodles according to package directions. Drain and keep warm.

2. Place green onion and green pepper in covered microwave-safe dish and microwave on high for 1 minute.

3. Add mushrooms and microwave for another minute, or until all vegetables are tender.

4. Add soup, Worcestershire sauce, Tabasco (if using), pimiento, olives, and milk and stir well. Microwave, covered, for 1–2 minutes, until mixture is hot and bubbly.

5. Add cooked shrimp and noodles and stir to mix. Microwave for 30 seconds to 1 minute, or until mixture is hot.

Eggplant and Tomato Stew

NUTRITIONAL ANALYSIS (per serving)

Calories: **135**   Protein: **4g**   Carbohydrates: **26g**   Fat: **3g**   Saturated Fat: **1g**   Cholesterol: **0mg**   Sodium: **22mg**
Fiber: **9g**   PCF Ratio: **12-69-19**   Exchange Approx.: **½ Fat, 4 Vegetables**

INGREDIENTS | SERVES 4

2 eggplants, trimmed but left whole

2 teaspoons olive oil

1 medium-sized Spanish onion, chopped

1 teaspoon chopped garlic

2 cups cooked or canned unsalted tomatoes, chopped, with liquid

Optional seasonings, to taste:

1 teaspoon hot pepper sauce

Ketchup

Nonfat plain yogurt

Fresh parsley sprigs

1. Preheat the oven to 400°F.

2. Roast eggplants on a baking sheet until soft, about 45 minutes. Remove all meat from eggplants.

3. In large sauté pan, heat the oil. Sauté the onions and garlic for approximately 2–3 minutes.

4. Add the eggplant and all the other ingredients, except the yogurt and parsley. Remove from heat and transfer to food processor; pulse until it becomes creamy.

5. Serve at room temperature, garnished with a dollop of yogurt and parsley, if desired.

CHAPTER 13

Pasta, Rice, Grains, and Beans

Quick Tomato Sauce

NUTRITIONAL ANALYSIS (per serving, without salt)

Calories: 40   Protein: 1g   Carbohydrates: 6g   Fat: 2g   Saturated Fat: 0g   Cholesterol: 0mg   Sodium: 10mg
Fiber: 1g   PCF Ratio: 9-49-42   Exchange Approx.: 1 Vegetable, ½ Fat

INGREDIENTS | SERVES 8

2 pounds very ripe tomatoes

2 tablespoons extra-virgin olive oil

2 cloves garlic, minced

½ teaspoon ground cumin

2 large sprigs fresh thyme, or ½ teaspoon dried thyme

1 bay leaf

Kosher or sea salt and freshly ground black pepper, to taste (optional)

3 tablespoons total of chopped fresh basil, oregano, tarragon, and parsley or cilantro, or a combination of all the listed herbs, to taste. If using dried herbs, reduce the amount to 1 tablespoon.

Remember . . .

The addition of ¼ teaspoon granulated sugar in tomato sauce helps cut the acidity of the tomatoes without affecting the Exchange Approximations for the recipe.

1. Peel and seed the tomatoes. Chop with a knife or food processor.

2. Heat a large skillet and add olive oil. Reduce heat to low and sauté garlic and cumin for 1 minute.

3. Add tomatoes, thyme, bay leaf, salt, and pepper, if using. If using dried herbs, add now. Simmer, uncovered, over medium heat for 8–10 minutes, stirring often. Reduce heat to maintain a simmer, if necessary. Simmer until tomatoes are soft and sauce has thickened, about 30 minutes.

4. Discard bay leaf and thyme sprigs and adjust seasoning to taste. If using fresh herbs, add just before serving.

Basic Tomato Sauce

NUTRITIONAL ANALYSIS (per serving, without salt)

Calories: 37   Protein: 1g   Carbohydrates: 5g   Fat: 2g   Saturated Fat: 0g   Cholesterol: 0mg   Sodium: 104 mg
Fiber: 1g   PCF Ratio: 9-55-36   Exchange Approx.: 1½ Vegetables

INGREDIENTS | YIELDS ABOUT 5 CUPS; SERVING SIZE: ¼ CUP

2 tablespoons olive oil

2 cups coarsely chopped yellow onion

½ cup sliced carrots

2 cloves garlic, minced

4 cups canned Italian plum tomatoes with juice

1 teaspoon dried oregano

1 teaspoon dried basil

¼ teaspoon sugar

Kosher or sea salt and freshly ground black pepper, to taste (optional)

Dash of ground anise seed (optional)

1. Heat olive oil in large, deep skillet or saucepan over medium-high heat. Add the onions, carrots, and garlic and sauté until onions are transparent, approximately 2–3 minutes. For a richer-tasting sauce, allow onions to caramelize or reach a light golden brown.)

2. Purée the tomatoes in a food processor.

3. Add the puréed tomatoes, oregano, basil, and sugar to the onion mixture along with salt, pepper, and anise, if using. Simmer, partially covered, for 45 minutes.

4. If you prefer a smoother sauce, process sauce in food processor again.

Culinary Antacids

Stir in 2 teaspoons Smucker's Low-Sugar Grape Jelly to tame hot chili or acidic sauces such as tomato sauce. You won't really notice the flavor of the jelly, and it will do a great job of reducing any tart, bitter, or acidic tastes in your sauce.

Fresh Garden Spaghetti Sauce

NUTRITIONAL ANALYSIS (per serving, without salt)

Calories: 81   Protein: 2g   Carbohydrates: 10g   Fat: 4g   Saturated Fat: 1g   Cholesterol: 0mg   Sodium: 33mg
Fiber: 2g   PCF Ratio: 9-49-42   Exchange Approx.: 2 Vegetables, 1 Fat

INGREDIENTS | SERVES 12

3 tablespoons olive oil

1 cup chopped celery

1 cup finely chopped onion

1 cup chopped green (or sweet red) pepper

2 cloves garlic, crushed

8 cups fresh tomatoes, peeled and crushed

1 (5½-ounce) can tomato paste

1 cup grated zucchini

1 tablespoon chopped fresh oregano

1 tablespoon chopped fresh basil

½ teaspoon crushed red pepper

½ cup dry red wine

Salt, to taste

1. In large, heavy saucepan or Dutch oven, heat the oil. Add the celery, onion, and peppers and sauté for 5 minutes. Add crushed garlic and sauté for an additional 2 minutes.

2. Add the crushed tomatoes, tomato paste, zucchini, oregano, basil, and red pepper. Bring to a boil. Reduce heat and simmer for 2–3 hours.

3. Add wine during last 30 minutes of cooking. Add salt to taste.

Tip

Don't waste unused tomato paste left in can. Spoon out tablespoon-sized portions and place on plastic wrap or in sandwich baggies. Seal packages and store in freezer. When you need tomato paste in a recipe, add frozen paste directly to sauce; no need to defrost.

Fusion Lo Mein

NUTRITIONAL ANALYSIS (per serving)

Calories: **126**   Protein: **5g**   Carbohydrates: **26g**   Fat: **1g**   Saturated Fat: **0g**   Cholesterol: **0mg**   Sodium: **35mg**
Fiber: **4g**   PCF Ratio: **14-77-9**   Exchange Approx.: **1 Starch, 1 Vegetable, ½ Fruit**

INGREDIENTS | SERVES 6

2 tablespoons rice vinegar

2 tablespoons thawed pineapple-orange juice concentrate

2 teaspoons minced shallots

2 teaspoons lemon juice

1 teaspoon cornstarch

1 teaspoon Worcestershire sauce (see recipe for homemade in Chapter 16)

1 teaspoon honey

2 cloves garlic, minced

1 teaspoon olive oil

¾ cup chopped green onions

1 cup diagonally sliced (¼" thick) carrots

1 cup julienned yellow bell pepper

1 cup julienned red bell pepper

3 cups small broccoli florets

1 cup fresh bean sprouts

1½ cups cooked pasta

1. In a food processor or blender, combine the vinegar, juice concentrate, shallots, lemon juice, cornstarch, Worcestershire, honey, and garlic. Process until smooth.

2. Heat a wok or large nonstick skillet coated with cooking spray over medium-high heat until hot. Then add the olive oil. Add the onions and stir-fry for 1 minute.

3. Add the carrots, bell peppers, and broccoli and stir-fry for 1 minute. Cover pan and cook for 2 more minutes.

4. Add the vinegar mixture and sprouts. Bring mixture to a boil and cook, uncovered, for 30 seconds, stirring constantly.

5. Add cooked pasta and toss to mix.

Roasted Butternut Squash Pasta

NUTRITIONAL ANALYSIS (per serving)

Calories: 216   Protein: 5g   Carbohydrates: 40g   Fat: 5g   Saturated Fat: 1g   Cholesterol: 0mg   Sodium: 8mg
Fiber: 2g   PCF Ratio: 9-70-21   Exchange Approx.: 2 Starches, 1 Fat, ½ Vegetable

INGREDIENTS | SERVES 4

1 butternut squash
4 teaspoons extra-virgin olive oil
1 clove garlic, minced
1 cup chopped red onion
2 teaspoons red wine vinegar
¼ teaspoon dried oregano
2 cups cooked pasta
Freshly ground black pepper (optional)

Tip

For added flavor, use roasted instead of raw garlic. Roasting garlic causes it to caramelize, adding a natural sweetness.

1. Preheat the oven to 400°F.

2. Cut squash in half and scoop out seeds.

3. Using nonstick spray, coat 1 side of 2 pieces of heavy-duty foil large enough to wrap squash halves. Wrap squash in foil; place on a baking sheet. Bake for 1 hour, or until tender.

4. Scoop out the baked squash flesh and discard the rind. Rough-chop the flesh.

5. Add olive oil, garlic, and onion to a nonstick skillet and sauté for about 5 minutes until onion is transparent. (Alternatively, put oil, garlic, and onion in covered microwave-safe dish and microwave on high for 2–3 minutes.)

6. Remove pan from heat and stir in the vinegar and oregano.

7. Add the squash and stir to coat in the onion mixture. Add pasta and toss to mix. Season with freshly ground black pepper, if desired.

Pasta with Artichokes

NUTRITIONAL ANALYSIS (per serving)

Calories: **308**   Protein: **10g**   Carbohydrates: **47g**   Fat: **9g**   Saturated Fat: **2g**   Cholesterol: **2mg**   Sodium: **87mg**
Fiber: **3g**   PCF Ratio: **13-60-27**   Exchange Approx.: **1 Medium-Fat Meat, 2 Vegetables, 1 Starch, 2 Fats**

INGREDIENTS | SERVES 4

1 (10-ounce) package frozen artichoke hearts

1¼ cups water

1 tablespoon lemon juice

4 teaspoons olive oil

2 cloves garlic, minced

¼ cup sundried tomatoes packed in oil, drained and chopped

¼ teaspoon red pepper flakes

2 teaspoons dried parsley

2 cups cooked pasta

¼ cup grated Parmesan cheese

Freshly ground black pepper, to taste (optional)

Tip

You can decrease the amount of water to 3 tablespoons and add it with the artichokes and lemon juice to a covered microwave-safe dish. Microwave according to package directions; reserve all liquid. This results in a stronger lemon flavor, which compensates for the lack of salt in this recipe.

1. Cook the artichokes in water and lemon juice according to package directions. Drain, reserving ¼ cup of liquid. Cool artichokes and then cut into quarters.

2. Heat olive oil in a nonstick skillet over medium heat. Add the garlic and sauté for 1 minute. Reduce heat to low.

3. Stir in the artichokes and tomatoes and simmer for 1 minute.

4. Stir in the reserved artichoke liquid, red pepper, and parsley and simmer for 5 minutes.

5. Pour artichoke sauce over the pasta in a large bowl. Toss gently to coat. Sprinkle with cheese and top with pepper, if desired.

Pasta with Creamed Clam Sauce

NUTRITIONAL ANALYSIS (per serving)

Calories: **226**   Protein: **15g**   Carbohydrates: **24g**   Fat: **7g**   Saturated Fat: **2g**   Cholesterol: **25mg**   Sodium: **209mg**
Fiber: **1g**   PCF Ratio: **27-43-30**   Exchange Approx.: **1 Lean Meat, 1 Starch, 1 Fat, ½ Skim Milk**

INGREDIENTS | SERVES 4

1 (6½-ounce) can chopped clams

4 teaspoons olive oil

1 clove garlic, minced

1 tablespoon dry white wine or dry vermouth

½ cup Mock Cream (see Chapter 16)

¼ cup freshly grated Parmesan cheese

2 cups cooked pasta

Freshly ground black pepper, to taste (optional)

1. Drain the clams, reserving the juice.

2. Heat the olive oil in a large nonstick skillet. Add the garlic and sauté for 1 minute.

3. Stir the clams into the skillet and sauté for 1 minute. With a slotted spoon, transfer the clams to a bowl and cover to keep warm.

4. Add the wine and reserved clam juice to the skillet. Bring to a boil and reduce by half, approximately 4–5 minutes.

5. Lower heat and add the mock cream. Cook for about 2–3 minutes, being careful not to boil the cream.

6. Stir in the Parmesan cheese and continue to heat for 1 minute, stirring constantly.

7. Add the pasta and toss with sauce. Divide into 4 equal servings. Serve immediately, topped with freshly ground pepper, if desired.

Whole-Grain Noodles with Caraway Cabbage

NUTRITIONAL ANALYSIS (per serving)

Calories: **169**   Protein: **6g**   Carbohydrates: **27g**   Fat: **5g**   Saturated Fat: **1g**   Cholesterol: **0mg**   Sodium: **250mg**

Fiber: **5g**   PCF Ratio: **14-60-26**   Exchange Approx.: **1 Starch, 1 Vegetable, 1 Fat**

INGREDIENTS | SERVES 6

2 tablespoons olive oil

½ cup chopped onion

2 cups coarsely chopped cabbage

1½ cups Brussels sprouts, trimmed and halved

2 teaspoons caraway seed

1½ cups low-sodium chicken broth

¼ teaspoon fresh ground pepper

¼ teaspoon salt

6 ounces whole-grain noodles

1. Heat the olive oil in a large saucepan. Add the onions and sauté for about 5 minutes until translucent.

2. Add the cabbage and Brussels sprouts and cook over medium heat for 3 minutes.

3. Stir in the caraway seed, broth, pepper, and salt. Cover and simmer for 5–8 minutes until the vegetables are crisp-tender.

4. Cook noodles in boiling water until tender. Drain.

5. Mix noodles and vegetables together in a large bowl and serve.

Tuscan Pasta Fagioli

NUTRITIONAL ANALYSIS (per serving)

Calories: **317**   Protein: **15g**   Carbohydrates: **54g**   Fat: **6g**   Saturated Fat: **1g**   Cholesterol: **2mg**   Sodium: **248mg**
Fiber: **11g**   PCF Ratio: **18-65-17**   Exchange Approx.: **3 Starches, ½ Vegetable, 1 Fat**

INGREDIENTS | SERVES 6

2 tablespoons olive oil

⅓ cup chopped onion

3 cloves garlic, minced

½ pound tomatoes, peeled and chopped

5 cups low-sodium vegetable stock

¼ teaspoon freshly ground pepper

3 cups cannellini beans, rinsed and drained

2½ cups whole-grain pasta shells

2 tablespoons Parmesan cheese

1. Heat the olive oil in large pot. Gently cook the onions and garlic until soft but not browned, approximately 2–3 minutes.

2. Add the tomatoes, vegetable stock, and pepper.

3. Purée 1½ cups of cannellini beans in a food processor or blender. Add to stock in pot. Cover and simmer for 20–30 minutes.

4. While stock is simmering, cook the pasta until al dente; and then drain. Add remaining beans and pasta to stock and heat through. Serve with Parmesan cheese.

Brown Rice and Vegetable Sauté

NUTRITIONAL ANALYSIS (per serving)

Calories: **154** Protein: **5g** Carbohydrates: **26g** Fat: **4g** Saturated Fat: **1g** Cholesterol: **0mg** Sodium: **352mg**
Fiber: **3g** PCF Ratio: **12-64-24** Exchange Approx.: **1 Starch, 1½ Vegetables, 1 Fat**

INGREDIENTS | SERVES 4

½ cup brown rice, uncooked
1 cup water
1 tablespoon olive oil
½ cup chopped onions
1 cup chopped red bell peppers
1 teaspoon minced garlic
4 ounces mushrooms, sliced
1 (12-ounce) package fresh bean sprouts
1 tablespoon reduced-sodium soy sauce
1 teaspoon grated fresh ginger

1. Add the rice to water and bring to a boil. Reduce heat, cover, and simmer for 35–40 minutes, until cooked.

2. In a large nonstick skillet or wok, heat the olive oil. Add the onions, red pepper, and garlic and cook until onion is translucent, approximately 2–3 minutes.

3. Add the mushrooms, bean sprouts, and soy sauce and cook on low heat for 3 minutes.

4. Add the rice and ginger and mix the ingredients. Cook on low for 2–3 minutes.

Squash and Bulgur Pilaf

NUTRITIONAL ANALYSIS (per serving)

Calories: **151**   Protein: **5g**   Carbohydrates: **22g**   Fat: **6g**   Saturated Fat: **1g**   Cholesterol: **0mg**   Sodium: **190mg**
Fiber: **5g**   PCF Ratio: **13-54-32**   Exchange Approx.: **1 Starch, ½ Vegetable, 2 Fats**

INGREDIENTS | SERVES 6

½ cup chopped onions

1 teaspoon minced garlic

1½ cups yellow summer squash, cut into ½" pieces

1 cup bulgur wheat

1 tablespoon olive oil

2 cups low-sodium chicken broth

½ teaspoon cinnamon

¼ cup dried currants

¼ cup chopped walnuts

1. In a large nonstick skillet, sauté the onions, garlic, yellow squash, and bulgur wheat in olive oil until the onions are tender, about 5 minutes.

2. Stir in the chicken broth and cinnamon. Heat to boiling. Reduce heat and simmer, covered, for 10 minutes.

3. Stir in the currants and continue to simmer for an additional 15 minutes. Add walnuts just before serving.

Herbed Quinoa with Sundried Tomatoes

NUTRITIONAL ANALYSIS (per serving)

Calories: **119**   Protein: **5g**   Carbohydrates: **21g**   Fat: **2g**   Saturated Fat: **0g**   Cholesterol: **0mg**   Sodium: **193mg**
Fiber: **2g**   PCF Ratio: **17-71-12**   Exchange Approx.: **1 Starch, ½ Very-Lean Meat, 2 Fat**

INGREDIENTS | SERVES 6

½ tablespoon olive oil

¼ cup chopped onion

1 clove minced garlic

1 cup quinoa

2 cups low-sodium chicken broth

½ cup sliced fresh mushrooms

6 sundried tomatoes, cut into ¼" pieces

1 teaspoon Italian-blend seasoning

Cooking Time for Quinoa

Quinoa takes no longer to cook than rice or pasta, usually about 15 minutes. You can tell quinoa is cooked when grains have turned from white to transparent, and the spiral-like germ has separated from the seed.

1. In a medium saucepan, heat the olive oil and sauté the onions and garlic, approximately 2–3 minutes.

2. Rinse the quinoa in very fine mesh strainer before cooking. Add quinoa and broth to the saucepan. Bring to a boil for 2 minutes.

3. Add the mushrooms, sundried tomatoes, and Italian seasoning.

4. Reduce heat and cover. Cook for 15 minutes, or until all water is absorbed.

Quinoa with Roasted Vegetables

NUTRITIONAL ANALYSIS (per serving)

Calories: 120   Protein: 4g   Carbohydrates: 9g   Fat: 4g   Saturated Fat: 0g   Cholesterol: 0mg   Sodium: 151mg   Fiber: 4g   PCF Ratio: 12-62-26   Exchange Approx.: 1 Starch, 1 Vegetable, 2 Fats

INGREDIENTS | SERVES 4

⅔ cup green pepper

½ cup red pepper (mildly hot variety)

3 cups eggplant, cut into 1" cubes

2 cloves garlic, finely chopped

1 tablespoon olive oil

½ teaspoon Texas Seasoning Blend (see Chapter 17)

¼ teaspoon cumin

½ cup quinoa

1 cup water

¼ teaspoon salt

Another Idea

Cook quinoa as outlined in steps 4 and 5. Combine with 3 cups of Oven-Roasted Ratatouille recipe found in Chapter 14. Nutritional Analysis for 1 cup serving: Calories: 162; Protein: 7g; Carbohydrates: 26g; Fat: 3g; Saturated Fat: 0g; Cholesterol: 1mg; Sodium: 202mg; Fiber: 4g; PCF Ratio: 13-69-18; Exchange Approx.: 1 Starch, 2 Vegetables, ½ Fat.

1. Preheat the oven to 375°F.

2. Combine the peppers, eggplant, garlic, olive oil, Texas Seasoning, and cumin in a 2-quart baking dish. Cover and roast for 20 minutes.

3. Remove the cover and continue to roast in the oven for about 30 minutes until vegetables are browned and cooked soft. Remove from oven and replace cover.

4. Rinse quinoa in very fine mesh strainer before cooking. Bring water and salt to a boil. Add quinoa and bring to a boil for 5 minutes. Cover, remove from heat, and let it stand for 15 minutes.

5. Once quinoa is cooked and all water is absorbed, add the roasted vegetables and serve.

Kasha-Stuffed Red Peppers

NUTRITIONAL ANALYSIS (per serving)

Calories: 383   Protein: 22g   Carbohydrates: 54g   Fat: 12g   Saturated Fat: 5g   Cholesterol: 40mg   Sodium: 387mg
Fiber: 11g   PCF Ratio: 22-53-25   Exchange Approx.: 2 Starches, 4 Vegetables, 1½ Lean Meats, 2 Fats

INGREDIENTS | SERVES 4

2 pounds red peppers (4 large)
1 cup kasha
1 egg white, lightly beaten
Nonstick cooking spray
2 cups low-sodium beef broth
4 ounces lean ground beef
1 cup finely chopped onion
5 ounces (½ package) frozen chopped spinach, thawed and drained
½ cup feta cheese, crumbled
½ cup canned diced tomatoes
1 teaspoon oregano
⅛ teaspoon crushed red pepper
1½ cups water

Save the Tomato Juice

Most canned tomatoes are packed in juice or puréed tomato. When you open a can, save juices and add to recipes when liquids are called for. In this recipe, tomato juice from the can could substitute some water used to cook peppers in.

1. Remove the tops and seeds of the red peppers and discard. Set remaining pepper "cups" aside.

2. Preheat the oven to 375°F.

3. Mix kasha and egg white together in a small bowl.

4. In a large nonstick saucepan sprayed with nonstick cooking spray, add kasha and cook over high heat for 2–3 minutes, stirring constantly, until the kasha kernels are separated.

5. Add the beef broth slowly. Reduce heat, cover, and cook for 7–10 minutes, until kasha kernels are tender. Transfer to a large bowl.

6. Brown the beef in a small nonstick skillet. Add onions and cook for 2–3 minutes, until slightly softened.

7. Add the beef mixture and chopped spinach to the cooked kasha and mix well. Stir in the feta cheese, diced tomato, oregano, and crushed red pepper. Divide mixture equally and stuff into each red pepper.

8. Place peppers in 9" × 9" baking dish. Pour water around the peppers.

9. Cover the dish with foil and bake for 60–75 minutes, or until peppers are cooked.

Red and White Bean Salad

NUTRITIONAL ANALYSIS (per serving)

Calories: 222   Protein: 8g   Carbohydrates: 27g   Fat: 10g   Saturated Fat: 1g   Cholesterol: 0mg   Sodium: 471mg
Fiber: 7g   PCF Ratio: 17-55-27   Exchange Approx.: 1½ Starches, 1 Vegetable, 1 Very-Lean Meat, 2 Fats

INGREDIENTS | SERVES 8

2 cups navy beans, cooked
2 cups red beans, cooked
1 cup chopped arugula
¼ cup lemon juice
3 tablespoons olive oil
¼ teaspoon fresh ground pepper
1 cup thinly sliced red onion
8 ounces cherry tomatoes, cut in half

1. Combine the beans together in a medium bowl.

2. Whisk together the arugula, lemon juice, olive oil, and pepper and pour over the beans.

3. Add the onions and toss lightly to mix. Refrigerate the mixture for at least 3 hours.

4. Just before serving, toss in the cherry tomatoes and mix lightly.

About Arugula

Arugula has several other names such as rocket, rugula, roquette, and rucola. It is sometimes found in baby greens or mesclun mixes. It has a nutty and peppery flavor, which can add interest to a salad or sandwich. Give arugula a try!

Zesty Black Bean Salsa

NUTRITIONAL ANALYSIS (per serving)

Calories: **86**   Protein: **3g**   Carbohydrates: **12g**   Fat: **3g**   Saturated Fat: **0g**   Cholesterol: **0mg**   Sodium: **125mg**
Fiber: **4g**   PCF Ratio: **15-53-32**   Exchange Approx.: **½ Starch, 1 Vegetable, 1 Fat**

INGREDIENTS | SERVES 10

1 cup chopped red onion
¼ cup chopped cilantro
¼ cup chopped parsley
1 small jalapeño pepper
1½ cups black beans, cooked
4 cups chopped tomatoes
3 tablespoons lime juice
2 tablespoons olive oil
Freshly ground black pepper

1. Place the onion, cilantro, parsley, and jalapeño in a food processor and finely chop.

2. In a medium bowl, combine the onion mixture, black beans, and tomatoes.

3. In a separate small bowl, whisk together the lime juice, olive oil, and fresh ground pepper. Pour over beans and mix well. Chill before serving.

Using Canned Beans Versus Cooking Your Own

Canned beans are very convenient and can save you time. Keep in mind the sodium content of recipes will be higher with canned beans. Reduce sodium content in canned beans by draining and thoroughly rinsing them with cold water before using.

Whole-Wheat Couscous Salad

NUTRITIONAL ANALYSIS (per serving)

Calories: 153   Protein: 4g   Carbohydrates: 15g   Fat: 9g   Saturated Fat: 1g   Cholesterol: 0mg   Sodium: 85mg
Fiber: 2g   PCF Ratio: 9-38-52   Exchange Approx.: 1 Starch, 2 Fats

INGREDIENTS | SERVES 8

1 cup low-sodium chicken broth

¼ cup dried currants

½ teaspoon cumin

¾ cup whole-wheat couscous

¼ cup olive oil

2 tablespoons lemon juice

1 cup broccoli, chopped and steamed to crisp-tender

3 tablespoons pine nuts

1 tablespoon chopped fresh parsley

Aren't Currants Just Small Raisins?

Dried currants may look like miniature raisins, but are actually quite different. Currants are berries from a shrub, not a vine, and there are red and black varieties. Black currants are rich in phytonutrients and antioxidants. They have twice the potassium of bananas and four times the vitamin C of oranges!

1. Combine the chicken broth, currants, and cumin in a medium saucepan and bring to a boil.

2. Remove from the heat and stir in the couscous. Cover and let sit until cool. Fluff couscous with fork 2 or 3 times during the cooling process.

3. In a small bowl, whisk together the olive oil and lemon juice.

4. Add the steamed broccoli and pine nuts to the couscous.

5. Pour oil and lemon juice over couscous and toss lightly. Garnish with chopped parsley.

CHAPTER 14

Vegetable Sides

Vegetable Broth

NUTRITIONAL ANALYSIS (per serving)

Calories: **10**   Protein: **0g**   Carbohydrates: **2g**   Fat: **0g**   Saturated Fat: **0g**   Cholesterol: **0mg**   Sodium: **8mg**
Fiber: **1g**   PCF Ratio: **11-85-4**   Exchange Approx.: **1 Free Vegetable**

INGREDIENTS | YIELDS ABOUT 2½ QUARTS; SERVING SIZE: ¾ CUP

4 carrots, peeled and chopped

2 celery stalks and leaves, chopped

1 green bell pepper, seeded and chopped

2 medium zucchini, chopped

1 small onion, chopped

1 cup chopped fresh spinach

2 cups chopped leeks

½ cup chopped scallions

1 cup chopped green beans

1 cup chopped parsnips

2 bay leaves

2 cloves garlic, crushed

Sea salt and freshly ground black pepper, to taste (optional)

3 quarts water

1. Place all of the ingredients in a large pot and bring to a boil.

2. Reduce heat, cover the pot, and simmer for 30 minutes, or until the vegetables are tender. Discard bay leaf.

3. Use a slotted spoon to transfer the vegetables to a different pot. Mix vegetables with some of the broth for a Free Exchange vegetable soup. Freeze the mixture in single-serving containers to keep on hand for a quick, heat-in-the-microwave snack.

4. Purée in blender or food processor and return to broth to add dietary fiber and body. Cool and freeze until needed.

Perpetual Broth

The easiest way to create vegetable broth is to keep a container in the freezer for saving liquid from cooked vegetables. Vegetable broth makes a great addition to sauces, soups, and many other recipes. Substitute it for meat broth in most recipes or use instead of water for cooking pasta, rice, and other grains.

Winter Vegetable Casserole

NUTRITIONAL ANALYSIS (per serving)

Calories: **218**   Protein: **5g**   Carbohydrates: **36g**   Fat: **7g**   Saturated Fat: **1g**   Cholesterol: **18mg**   Sodium: **392mg**
Fiber: **5g**   PCF Ratio: **9-64-27**   Exchange Approx.: **1½ Starches, 1½ Vegetables, 1 Fat**

INGREDIENTS | SERVES 6

Cooking spray
3 tablespoons butter
3 tablespoons all-purpose flour
½ teaspoon salt
¼ teaspoon white pepper
1½ cups low-fat milk
1½ potatoes, thinly sliced
1½ sweet potatoes, thinly sliced
1 cup peeled and sliced parsnips
1 cup sliced turnips
½ cup chopped onions

1. Preheat the oven to 350°F. Spray a 2-quart casserole dish with cooking spray.

2. In a small saucepan, melt the butter. Add the flour, salt, and pepper to make a roux. Gradually stir in the milk, cooking over low heat; stir well with wire whisk.

3. Bring milk to a boil, stirring constantly, until milk has thickened into a sauce, about 10 minutes. Remove from heat.

4. Arrange half of sliced vegetables in the casserole dish. Top with half of the chopped onion and half of the white sauce. Repeat to make a second layer.

5. Cover and cook for 45 minutes. Uncover and continue to cook until all vegetables are tender, about 60–70 minutes.

6. Let casserole stand 10 minutes before serving.

Healthy Onion Rings

NUTRITIONAL ANALYSIS (per serving, without salt)

Calories: 111 Protein: 4g Carbohydrates: 22g Fat: 1g Saturated Fat: 0g Cholesterol: 1mg Sodium: 255mg
Fiber: 1g PCF Ratio: 16-80-4 Exchange Approx.: 1 Vegetable, 1 Starch

INGREDIENTS | SERVES 4

1 cup yellow onion slices (¼" thick)
½ cup flour
½ cup nonfat plain yogurt
½ cup bread crumbs
Sea salt and freshly ground black pepper, to taste (optional)

1. Preheat the oven to 350°F.

2. Dredge the onion slices in flour and shake off any excess.

3. Dip onions in yogurt and dredge through the bread crumbs.

4. Prepare baking sheet with nonstick cooking spray. Arrange onion rings on pan and bake for 15–20 minutes.

5. Place under the broiler for an additional 2 minutes to brown. Season with salt and pepper, if desired.

Oven-Baked Red Potatoes

NUTRITIONAL ANALYSIS (per serving)

Calories: **120**   Protein: **2g**   Carbohydrates: **26g**   Fat: **1g**   Saturated Fat: **0g**   Cholesterol: **0g**   Sodium: **587mg**
Fiber: **2g**   PCF Ratio: **7-84-9**   Exchange Approx.: **1 Starch**

INGREDIENTS | SERVES 4

1 pound (16 ounces) small red potatoes, halved

¼ cup fresh lemon juice

1 teaspoon olive oil

1 teaspoon sea salt

¼ teaspoon freshly ground pepper

Remember the Roasting "Rack"

Use caution when roasting potatoes with meat: Potatoes will act like a sponge, soaking up fat. Your best option is to use lean cuts of meat and elevate them and vegetables above the fat by putting them on a roasting rack in a pan or making a "bridge" with celery to elevate meat. Discard celery when done.

1. Preheat the oven to 350°F.

2. Arrange the potatoes in a 13" × 9" ovenproof casserole dish.

3. In a small bowl, combine the remaining ingredients and then pour over the potatoes.

4. Bake for 30–40 minutes, or until potatoes are tender, turning 3–4 times to baste.

Broccoli Raab with Pine Nuts

NUTRITIONAL ANALYSIS (per serving)

Calories: 110   Protein: 5g   Carbohydrates: 6g   Fat: 8g   Saturated Fat: 1g   Cholesterol: 0mg   Sodium: 229mg
Fiber: 4g   PCF Ratio: 18-20-62   Exchange Approx.: 1 Vegetable, 1 Fat

INGREDIENTS | SERVES 4

¾ pound broccoli raab, cooked

1 tablespoon olive oil

4 cloves garlic, chopped

¼ cup sundried tomatoes, chopped

2 tablespoons pine nuts

¼ teaspoon salt

¼ teaspoon crushed red pepper

Preventing Bitter Broccoli Raab

Broccoli raab and other leafy greens (mustard or collard greens) can have a bitter taste once cooked. Rather than add extra salt to offset bitterness, this recipe calls for blanching for 2 minutes, which helps reduce bitterness. Blanching should be done as quickly as possible by starting with water at a full rolling boil, then removing after 2 minutes of boiling. If allowed to cook too long, the boiling process will reduce the amount of water-soluble nutrients found in the vegetables.

1. Prepare and blanch broccoli before beginning recipe: Rinse well and trim stems. Loosely chop leafy parts, then blanch in 2 quarts boiling water for 2 minutes. Drain well.

2. Heat the olive oil in a large skillet and add the garlic. Sauté the garlic for 1–2 minutes. Add cooked broccoli raab. Toss garlic and raab together well, so that oil and garlic are mixed evenly.

3. Add remaining ingredients and cook for an additional 2–3 minutes, until broccoli raab is tender.

Sweet Potato Crisps

NUTRITIONAL ANALYSIS (per serving, without salt)

Calories: **89**   Protein: **1g**   Carbohydrates: **16g**   Fat: **2g**   Saturated Fat: **1g**   Cholesterol: **0mg**   Sodium: **7mg**
Fiber: **9g**   PCF Ratio: **6-70-24**   Exchange Approx.: **1 Starch, ½ Fat**

INGREDIENTS | SERVES 2

1 small sweet potato or yam
1 teaspoon olive oil
Sea salt and freshly ground black pepper, to taste (optional)

1. Preheat the oven to 400°F.

2. Scrub the sweet potato and pierce the flesh several times with fork. Place on a microwave-safe plate and microwave for 5 minutes on high. Remove from microwave and wrap in aluminum foil. Set aside for 5 minutes.

3. Remove the foil. Peel the potato and cut into French fries.

4. Spread on a baking sheet treated with nonstick spray and spritz with olive oil. Bake for 10–15 minutes, or until crisp. There's a risk that sweet potato strips will caramelize and burn so check them often while cooking to ensure this doesn't occur. Lower oven temperature, if necessary.

5. Season with salt and pepper, if desired.

Sweet Potatoes with Onions and Apple

NUTRITIONAL ANALYSIS (per serving)

Calories: **127** Protein: **2g** Carbohydrates: **28g** Fat: **1g** Saturated Fat: **0g** Cholesterol: **1mg** Sodium: **144mg**
Fiber: **4g** PCF Ratio: **6-85-9** Exchange Approx.: **1 Starch, ½ Vegetable**

INGREDIENTS | **SERVES 6**

1 pound sweet potatoes (about 2 large)
½ teaspoon canola oil
1 cup thinly sliced onion
1 apple, peeled and chopped
½ cup low-sodium chicken broth

1. Wash and dry the sweet potatoes. Pierce the skins several times with a fork. Microwave on high for 5–8 minutes, or until tender. Allow to cool.

2. While sweet potatoes are cooling, heat the oil in a large nonstick skillet over medium-high heat. Add the onions and sauté until golden brown, about 10 minutes.

3. Add the chopped apple and chicken broth and cook until the onions are tender and have caramelized.

4. Scoop cooked sweet potatoes from skins into a microwaveable dish and mash lightly. Cover and microwave on high for 1–2 minutes, or until potatoes are heated. Top with sautéed onions and serve.

French Tarragon Green Beans

NUTRITIONAL ANALYSIS (per serving, without salt)

Calories: **59**   Protein: **0g**   Carbohydrates: **5g**   Fat: **3g**   Saturated Fat: **1g**   Cholesterol: **11mg**   Sodium: **105mg**
Fiber: **1g**   PCF Ratio: **3-32-65**   Exchange Approx.: **1 Vegetable, 1 Fat**

INGREDIENTS | SERVES 4

1½ tablespoons butter
¼ cup chopped red onion
½ pound fresh green beans
1 tablespoon finely chopped tarragon

1. Melt the butter in a nonstick pan. Add the onions and sauté until translucent, approximately 2–3 minutes.

2. Add the green beans. Cover and steam for 2–3 minutes.

3. Add tarragon and combine well. Steam for an additional 2–3 minutes.

Oven-Roasted Ratatouille

NUTRITIONAL ANALYSIS (per serving)

Calories: 87   Protein: 2g   Carbohydrates: 11g   Fat: 5g   Saturated Fat: 1g   Cholesterol: 0mg   Sodium: 452mg
Fiber: 3g   PCF Ratio: 9-46-46   Exchange Approx.: 2 Vegetables, 1 Fat

INGREDIENTS | SERVES 12

5 cups eggplant, peeled and cut into ½" cubes

3 cups yellow squash, cut into ½" pieces

½ pound green beans

½ cup chopped celery

1 cup chopped red onion

4 cloves garlic, chopped

1 (28-ounce) can diced tomatoes

1 tablespoon chopped fresh parsley

¼ teaspoon salt

½ teaspoon rosemary

½ teaspoon thyme

¼ cup olive oil

2 tablespoons balsamic vinegar

1. Preheat the oven to 375°F.

2. In a large Dutch oven or 9" × 13" baking dish, combine the eggplant, yellow squash, green beans, celery, onion, garlic, tomatoes, parsley, salt, rosemary, thyme, and olive oil.

3. Roast uncovered in oven. Stir after 30 minutes, then continue roasting for another 30 minutes, or until vegetables are softened and lightly browned on top.

4. Remove from oven. Stir in balsamic vinegar and serve.

Spaghetti Squash and Vegetable Mix

NUTRITIONAL ANALYSIS (per serving)

Calories: **127**   Protein: **4g**   Carbohydrates: **16g**   Fat: **6g**   Saturated Fat: **3g**   Cholesterol: **5mg**   Sodium: **169mg**
Fiber: **2g**   PCF Ratio: **12-47-41**   Exchange Approx.: **1 Starch, 1 Fat**

INGREDIENTS | SERVES 6

2 pounds spaghetti squash
Cooking spray
1 cup peas, fresh or frozen
2 tablespoons butter
8 ounces cherry tomatoes, cut in half
1 ounce grated Romano cheese
¼ teaspoon fresh ground pepper

Pasta Alternative

Spaghetti squash is a wonderful alternative to pasta because it is packed with vitamins, minerals, and fiber. While it has a consistency similar to spaghetti, it is much lower in carbohydrates: 1 cup of cooked spaghetti squash has 15g of carbohydrate, while 1 cup of cooked spaghetti has approximately 45g!

1. Preheat the oven to 400°F.

2. Cut the spaghetti squash in half and scoop out seeds. Spray a 9" × 13" baking dish with cooking spray and place the squash halves face down. Bake for 45 minutes, or until squash is soft-cooked.

3. When the squash is cool enough to handle, use a fork to scoop out cooked squash from the outer shell. Scoop into a medium-sized microwaveable bowl.

4. In a separate small saucepan, lightly steam peas for 2–3 minutes. Add to squash, along with butter, and mix well.

5. Place covered bowl in microwave and cook on high for 2–3 minutes.

6. Add cherry tomato halves and top with Romano cheese and pepper before serving.

Sesame Snap Peas

NUTRITIONAL ANALYSIS (per serving)

Calories: 49   Protein: 0g   Carbohydrates: 3g   Fat: 4g   Saturated Fat: 0g   Cholesterol: 0mg   Sodium: 149mg
Fiber: 2g   PCF Ratio: 2-27-72   Exchange Approx.: 1 Vegetable, ½ Fat

INGREDIENTS | SERVES 4

½ tablespoon canola oil
10 ounces fresh snap peas
¼ cup scallions, thinly sliced
1 tablespoon fresh grated ginger
2 teaspoons sesame oil
1 tablespoon sesame seeds

1. Heat the canola oil in a large nonstick skillet or wok.

2. Add the snap peas, scallions, and ginger and stir-fry until peas are crisp-tender, approximately 3–4 minutes.

3. Stir in the sesame oil and sesame seeds. Toss lightly and serve.

Amish-Style Turnips

NUTRITIONAL ANALYSIS (per serving)

Calories: 80   Protein: 2g   Carbohydrates: 12g   Fat: 3g   Saturated Fat: 2g   Cholesterol: 40mg   Sodium: 49mg
Fiber: 2g   PCF Ratio: 10-56-34   Exchange Approx.: 1 Vegetable, ½ Starch, ½ Fat

INGREDIENTS | SERVES 6

3 cups turnips, cooked and mashed
½ cup water
1 slice whole-wheat bread
1 tablespoon butter, melted
2 tablespoons Splenda Brown Sugar Blend
½ cup low-fat milk
1 egg

1. Preheat the oven to 375°F.

2. Cook turnips in advance. If using fresh turnips, wash, peel, and cut into 1" cubes. Put in covered dish with ½ cup water; microwave on high for 10–15 minutes, until tender.

3. Place the bread in a food processor. Using the pulse setting, process until bread is the consistency of fine bread crumbs.

4. In a medium bowl, mix together the bread crumbs, melted butter, Splenda, milk, and egg. Add the cooked turnip and mix well.

5. Turn mixture into a greased casserole dish. Bake uncovered for 30–35 minutes.

Greens in Garlic with Pasta

NUTRITIONAL ANALYSIS (per serving, without salt)

Calories: **176** Protein: **8g** Carbohydrates: **26g** Fat: **5g** Saturated Fat: **1g** Cholesterol: **0mg** Sodium: **17mg**
Fiber: **3g** PCF Ratio: **17-58-25** Exchange Approx.: **1 Free Vegetable, 1 Fat, 1 Starch, ½ Lean Meat**

INGREDIENTS | SERVES 4

2 teaspoons olive oil

4 cloves garlic, crushed

6 cups tightly packed loose-leaf greens (baby mustard, turnip, chard)

2 cups cooked pasta

2 teaspoons extra-virgin olive oil

¼ cup freshly grated Parmesan cheese

Salt and freshly ground black pepper, to taste (optional)

Sweet or Salty?

In most cases, when you add a pinch (less than ⅛ teaspoon) of sugar to a recipe, you can reduce the amount of salt without noticing a difference. Sugar acts as a flavor enhancer and magnifies the effect of the salt.

1. Place a sauté pan over medium heat. When hot, add 2 teaspoons of olive oil and garlic. Cook, stirring frequently, until golden brown, about 3–5 minutes, being careful not to burn garlic, as that makes it bitter.

2. Add the greens and sauté until coated in garlic oil, approximately 3–5 minutes. Remove from heat.

3. In large serving bowl, add pasta, cooked greens, 2 teaspoons of extra-virgin olive oil, and Parmesan cheese. Toss to mix. Serve immediately, and season as desired.

Vegetable Frittata (with Egg Substitute)

NUTRITIONAL ANALYSIS (per serving)

Calories: 171   Protein: 12g   Carbohydrates: 11g   Fat: 9g   Saturated Fat: 4g   Cholesterol: 195mg   Sodium: 252mg
Fiber: 2g   PCF Ratio: 28-24-48   Exchange Approx.: 1 Vegetable, 1 Lean Meat, 2½ Fats

INGREDIENTS | SERVES 4

1½ tablespoons olive oil

4 ounces red pepper, chopped

3 large eggs

4 ounces egg substitute (or egg whites)

½ cup asparagus, cut diagonally in 1" pieces

¾ cup potatoes, cooked and cubed

⅓ cup feta cheese, crumbled

1 teaspoon oregano

1. Preheat the oven to 350°F.

2. In an ovenproof nonstick skillet, heat the olive oil over medium heat. Add red peppers and cook until softened, approximately 3–4 minutes.

3. In a medium bowl, beat together the eggs and egg substitute. Add asparagus, potatoes, feta, and oregano and mix well.

4. Pour the egg mixture into the skillet. Gently stir until the eggs on bottom of pan begin to set. Gently pull cooked eggs from side of skillet, allowing liquid uncooked egg on top to come in contact with heated skillet. Repeat, working all around skillet, until most of eggs on top have begun to set.

5. Transfer skillet to oven and bake until top is set and dry to the touch, about 3–5 minutes.

6. Loosen the frittata around the edges of the skillet and invert onto a serving plate.

Crustless Zucchini and Artichoke Quiche

NUTRITIONAL ANALYSIS (per serving)

Calories: **224**   Protein: **24g**   Carbohydrates: **9g**   Fat: **10g**   Saturated Fat: **4g**   Cholesterol: **134mg**   Sodium: **798mg**
Fiber: **3g**   PCF Ratio: **43-16-41**   Exchange Approx.: **1 Vegetable, 1½ Lean Meats, 1½ Fats**

INGREDIENTS | SERVES 4

Nonstick cooking spray
1 tablespoon olive oil
¼ cup chopped onions
¾ cup grated zucchini
1 cup canned artichoke hearts, cut in ½" pieces
1½ cups light Cheddar cheese, grated
2 eggs
½ cup egg whites
½ cup fat-free cottage cheese
¼ teaspoon cayenne
¼ teaspoon salt
⅛ teaspoon fresh-ground pepper

1. Preheat the oven to 375°F. Spray a 9" pie plate with cooking spray.

2. In a large nonstick skillet, heat the olive oil. Add the onion and sauté until translucent, approximately 2–3 minutes.

3. Add the zucchini and artichoke hearts and cook for 3 minutes.

4. Sprinkle the grated cheese in the bottom of the pie plate. Add cooked vegetables on top of cheese.

5. In a small bowl, whisk the eggs, egg whites, cottage cheese, cayenne, salt, and pepper together. Pour over the vegetables.

6. Bake in oven for 35–40 minutes.

CHAPTER 15

Salads

Minted Lentil and Tomato Salad

NUTRITIONAL ANALYSIS (per serving)

Calories: 136   Protein: 4g   Carbohydrates: 11g   Fat: 9g   Saturated Fat: 1g   Cholesterol: 0mg   Sodium: 211mg
Fiber: 4g   PCF Ratio: 10-31-59   Exchange Approx.: ½ Starch, 1 Vegetable, ½ Lean Meat, 2 Fats

INGREDIENTS | SERVES 6

1 cup dry lentils
2 cups water
½ cup chopped onion
2 teaspoons minced garlic
¼ cup chopped celery
½ cup chopped green pepper
½ cup finely chopped parsley
2 tablespoons finely chopped fresh mint, or 2 teaspoons dried
¼ cup lemon juice
¼ cup olive oil
½ teaspoon salt
1 cup diced fresh tomato

1. Place the lentils and water in a medium-sized saucepan and bring to a quick boil. Reduce heat, cover, and cook on low for 15–20 minutes, or until tender. Drain and transfer to a medium bowl.

2. Add the onion, garlic, celery, green pepper, parsley, and mint and mix well.

3. In a small bowl, whisk together the lemon juice, olive oil, and salt. Pour into lentils and mix well. Cover and refrigerate for several hours.

4. Before serving, mix in the diced tomatoes.

Marinated Roasted Peppers and Eggplant

NUTRITIONAL ANALYSIS (per serving)

Calories: 179   Protein: 2g   Carbohydrates: 14g   Fat: 14g   Saturated Fat: 2g   Cholesterol: 0mg   Sodium: 5mg
Fiber: 6g   PCF Ratio: 5-29-66   Exchange Approx.: 3 Vegetables, 3 Fats

INGREDIENTS | SERVES 4

1 pound roasted red peppers

1 large eggplant, sliced into ¼"-thick rounds

2 tablespoons olive oil

1 tablespoon balsamic vinegar

2 tablespoons olive oil

1 tablespoon finely chopped onion

1 teaspoon oregano

Fresh ground pepper, to taste

Variations

You can use zucchini or yellow squash in place of eggplant. Other herb choices for the marinade include basil, thyme, or savory. Use marinated vegetables on top of tossed salads or grilled London broil.

1. Follow the procedure for roasting red peppers described in the Roasted Red Pepper and Plum Sauce recipe in Chapter 16. Set aside.

2. Brush eggplant slices with 2 tablespoons of olive oil. Place on preheated grill. Grill for about 5 minutes on each side until softened. Remove from grill and place in a container. Add roasted peppers to the container.

3. In a small bowl, prepare the marinade by whisking together the balsamic vinegar, 2 tablespoons olive oil, chopped onion, oregano, and pepper. Pour over vegetables. Cover and refrigerate for at least 3 hours before serving.

Spinach Salad with Pomegranate

NUTRITIONAL ANALYSIS (per serving)

Calories: 107   Protein: 4g   Carbohydrates: 8g   Fat: 8g   Saturated Fat: 1g   Cholesterol: 0mg   Sodium: 259mg
Fiber: 3g   PCF Ratio: 13-26-61   Exchange Approx.: 1 Vegetable, 2 Fats

INGREDIENTS | SERVES 6

1 pound fresh spinach

½ cup very thinly sliced red onion

8 ounces fresh tomatoes, cut into ½"
wedges

⅓ cup chopped walnuts

½ teaspoon salt

¼ cup lemon juice

1½ tablespoons olive oil

¼ cup pomegranate seeds

1. Wash the spinach thoroughly and drain well. Loosely chop and place in a large bowl.

2. Add the onions, tomato, and walnuts and toss lightly.

3. In a small bowl, whisk together the salt, lemon juice, and olive oil. Drizzle over salad and toss lightly.

4. Garnish salad with pomegranate seeds.

For a Different Twist: Toasted Almond Seasoning

Add an extra flavor dimension to salads, rice dishes, or vegetables by sprinkling toasted almonds over the top. Toast ½ cup ground raw almonds in a nonstick skillet over low heat, stirring frequently, until they are a light brown color. Store the cooled almonds in an airtight container in a cool, dry place. This low-sodium substitute has only 16 calories per teaspoon, a PCF Ratio of 14-12-74, and counts as a ½ Fat Exchange Approximation.

Tabbouleh

NUTRITIONAL ANALYSIS (per serving)

Calories: 144   Protein: 3g   Carbohydrates: 15g   Fat: 9g   Saturated Fat: 1g   Cholesterol: 0mg   Sodium: 212mg
Fiber: 4g   PCF Ratio: 7-38-55   Exchange Approx.: ½ Starch, 1 Vegetable, 2 Fats

INGREDIENTS | SERVES 6

1 cup boiling water
½ cup bulgur wheat
1 cup fresh parsley, packed and finely chopped
⅓ cup fresh mint, finely chopped
½ cup finely chopped red onion
1 cup chopped cucumber
¼ cup lemon juice
¼ cup olive oil
½ teaspoon salt
Freshly ground pepper, to taste
1 cup chopped fresh tomato
2 cups leaf lettuce (optional)

1. In a small bowl, pour boiling water over bulgur wheat. Let stand for 20 minutes.

2. When bulgur is softened, drain and squeeze out any excess water using a colander lined with cheesecloth.

3. In a medium bowl, combine the parsley, mint, onion, cucumber, and wheat.

4. Add the lemon juice, olive oil, salt, and ground pepper and mix well.

5. Cover and refrigerate for at least 3 hours.

6. Just before serving, add chopped tomatoes and toss lightly. Serve as is or on bed of leaf lettuce.

Parsley . . . Not Just a Garnish

Parsley is a key ingredient in tabbouleh and many other Middle Eastern dishes. Parsley is low in calories and packed with vitamin C, iron, and other trace minerals. Add it liberally to all salads.

Tomato and Cucumber Salad with Mint

NUTRITIONAL ANALYSIS (per serving)

Calories: 68   Protein: 1g   Carbohydrates: 7g   Fat: 5g   Saturated Fat: 1g   Cholesterol: 0mg   Sodium: 202mg   Fiber: 1g   PCF Ratio: 5-32-63   Exchange Approx.: 1 Vegetable, 1 Fat

INGREDIENTS | SERVES 6

2 cucumbers
⅓ cup red wine vinegar
1 teaspoon sugar
½ teaspoon salt
2 cups chopped tomatoes
⅔ cup chopped red onion
¼ cup chopped fresh mint
2 tablespoons olive oil

1. Cut cucumbers into ½"-wide pieces. Place in a medium bowl.

2. Add the vinegar, sugar, and salt to the bowl and stir. Let stand at room temperature for 15 minutes.

3. Add the tomatoes, red onion, mint, and olive oil. Toss lightly to blend.

Cucumbers with Minted Yogurt

NUTRITIONAL ANALYSIS (per serving)

Calories: 31   Protein: 2g   Carbohydrates: 4g   Fat: 1g   Saturated Fat: 0g   Cholesterol: 2mg   Sodium: 52mg   Fiber: 1g   PCF Ratio: 27-56-17   Exchange Approx.: 1 Vegetable

INGREDIENTS | SERVES 8

1 cup nonfat plain yogurt
1 clove garlic, finely chopped
¼ teaspoon cumin
1 teaspoon lemon zest
½ cup mint
1 tablespoon lemon juice
¼ teaspoon salt
4 cups cucumbers, seeded and chopped

1. Combine the yogurt, garlic, cumin, lemon zest, mint, lemon juice, and salt in a blender or food processor. Blend until smooth.

2. Add the yogurt mixture to the cucumbers and mix. Chill before serving.

Tomatoes Stuffed with Quinoa Salad

NUTRITIONAL ANALYSIS (per serving)

Calories: **180**   Protein: **5g**   Carbohydrates: **24g**   Fat: **9g**   Saturated Fat: **2g**   Cholesterol: **4mg**   Sodium: **78mg**
Fiber: **4g**   PCF Ratio: **11-49-40**   Exchange Approx.: **½ Starch, 2½ Vegetables, 2½ Fats**

INGREDIENTS | SERVES 6

½ cup quinoa
1 cup water
6 large (3 pounds) tomatoes
1½ cups cucumber, peeled and finely diced
⅓ cup chopped fresh parsley
¼ cup chopped fresh mint
½ cup finely chopped red onion
3 tablespoons feta cheese, crumbled
2 tablespoons lemon juice
3 tablespoons olive oil

1. Rinse quinoa in a fine mesh strainer before cooking. To cook: Place quinoa and water in small saucepan and bring to a boil. Reduce heat, cover, and cook until all water is absorbed, about 15 minutes. Let cool.

2. Prepare the tomatoes: remove the caps and hollow out, leaving shell about ½" thick.

3. In a mixing bowl, combine the quinoa, cucumbers, parsley, mint, red onion, and feta cheese.

4. In a small bowl, mix the lemon juice and olive oil together. Pour over the quinoa and vegetables.

5. Stuff tomatoes with mixture and serve.

Wilted Lettuce with a Healthier Difference

NUTRITIONAL ANALYSIS (per serving)

Calories: 71   Protein: 2g   Carbohydrates: 7g   Fat: 5g   Saturated Fat: 1g   Cholesterol: 0mg   Sodium: 9mg
Fiber: 2g   PCF Ratio: 8-34-57   Exchange Approx.: 2 Free Vegetables, 1 Fat

INGREDIENTS | SERVES 1

½ teaspoon olive oil

¼ cup chopped red onion

1½ cups tightly packed loose-leaf lettuce

¼ teaspoon lemon juice or your choice of vinegar

½ teaspoon extra-virgin olive oil, walnut oil, or almond oil

Optional seasonings to taste:

Dried herbs of your choice, such as thyme or parsley

Pinch of sugar

Pinch of toasted sesame seeds or grated Parmesan cheese

1. In a heated nonstick skillet treated with nonstick spray, add ½ teaspoon of olive oil and all the red onion. Sauté until the onion is almost transparent, approximately 2–3 minutes.

2. Add the greens. Sauté greens until warmed and wilted, approximately 2 minutes.

3. In a salad bowl, whisk the lemon juice with ½ teaspoon oil. Add pinch of herbs and sugar, if using, and whisk into oil mixture.

4. Add the wilted greens to the salad bowl and toss with dressing. Top salad with pinch of toasted sesame seeds or Parmesan cheese, if desired. Serve immediately.

Adventuresome Additions

Dried cranberries or other dried fruit are delicious in wilted lettuce dishes; the addition of diced apples or pineapple makes a perfect wilted greens accompaniment for pork.

Mandarin Snap Pea Salad

NUTRITIONAL ANALYSIS (per serving, without dressing):

Calories: **76** Protein: **4g** Carbohydrates: **16g** Fat: **0g** Saturated Fat: **0g** Cholesterol: **0mg** Sodium: **344mg**
Fiber: **4g** PCF Ratio: **19-78-3** Exchange Approx.: ½ Starch, 1 Vegetable, ½ Lean Meat, ½ Fat

INGREDIENTS | SERVES 8

¾ pound snap peas, cut into ½" pieces

1 cup canned mandarin oranges, drained

1½ cups canned kidney beans, rinsed and drained

1 cup thinly sliced red onion

½ cup chopped fresh parsley

2 cups chopped cabbage

⅓ cup poppy seed dressing (see recipe in sidebar)

1. In a medium bowl, combine the snap peas, mandarin oranges, kidney beans, onions, parsley, and cabbage.

2. Mix in the poppy seed dressing. Refrigerate several hours before serving.

Poppy Seed Dressing

Combine ½ cup red wine vinegar, ¼ cup orange juice, 3 tablespoons lemon juice, ½ cup canola oil, 1 teaspoon Splenda Brown Sugar Blend, 1 teaspoon dry mustard, 1 teaspoon salt, and 1 tablespoon poppy seeds; mix well in covered jar. Store in refrigerator. Nutritional Analysis 1 ounce serving (1½ tablespoons): 68 Calories; Protein: 0g; Carbohydrates: 2g; Fat: 8g; Saturated Fat: 1g; Cholesterol: 0mg; Sodium: 79mg; PCF Ration: 1-8-91; Exchange Approx.: 1½ Fats

Broccoli-Cauliflower Slaw

NUTRITIONAL ANALYSIS (per serving)

Calories: 117 Protein: 6g Carbohydrates: 13g Fat: 5g Saturated Fat: 1g Cholesterol: 0mg Sodium: 46mg
Fiber: 1g PCF Ratio: 19-42-39 Exchange Approx.: 1 Misc. Carbohydrate, 1 Fat

INGREDIENTS | SERVES 8

4 cups raw broccoli florets

4 cups raw cauliflower

½ cup real mayonnaise

1 cup cottage cheese, 1% fat

3 tablespoons tarragon vinegar

1 tablespoon balsamic vinegar

⅛ cup packed brown sugar

3 tablespoons minced red onion

1. Put the broccoli and cauliflower in a food processor. Pulse-process until the consistency of shredded cabbage. Pour into a bowl.

2. Place remaining ingredients in the food processor and process until smooth. Pour resulting dressing over broccoli-cauliflower mixture and stir. Chill until ready to serve.

Tip

Substituting cottage cheese for some mayonnaise cuts fat and calories considerably. Cut them even more by using nonfat cottage cheese and mayonnaise.

Zesty Feta and Olive Salad

NUTRITIONAL ANALYSIS (per serving)

Calories: **109**   Protein: **3g**   Carbohydrates: **6g**   Fat: **8g**   Saturated Fat: **3g**   Cholesterol: **132mg**   Sodium: **326mg**
Fiber: **2g**   PCF Ratio: **11-22-66**   Exchange Approx.: **1** Vegetable, **2** Fats

INGREDIENTS | SERVES 4

2 ounces crumbled feta

1 small red onion, diced

½ cup chopped celery

½ cup diced cucumber

1 clove garlic, minced

1 teaspoon lemon zest

1 teaspoon orange zest

1 cup halved very small cherry tomatoes

½ cup mix of green and kalamata olives, pitted and sliced

1 tablespoon extra-virgin olive oil

2 tablespoons minced fresh Italian parsley

2 teaspoons minced fresh oregano

1 teaspoon minced fresh mint

1 tablespoon minced fresh cilantro (optional)

Large romaine or butter lettuce leaves

Freshly ground black pepper, to taste

1. In a large bowl, add the feta, onion, celery, cucumber, garlic, lemon zest, orange zest, tomatoes, and olives and mix.

2. Add the olive oil and fresh herbs and toss again.

3. Arrange lettuce leaves on 4 salad plates. Spoon the feta salad on top. Top with pepper and serve.

Avocado and Peach Salad

NUTRITIONAL ANALYSIS (per serving, without salt)

Calories: **160**   Protein: **2g**   Carbohydrates: **15g**   Fat: **11g**   Saturated Fat: **2g**   Cholesterol: **0mg**   Sodium: **11mg**
Fiber: **4g**   PCF Ratio: **6-35-59**   Exchange Approx.: **3 Fats, 1 Vegetable, ½ Fruit**

INGREDIENTS | SERVES 4

⅛ cup water
⅛ cup frozen orange juice concentrate
1 clove garlic, crushed
1 teaspoon rice wine vinegar
1 tablespoon extra-virgin olive oil
½ teaspoon vanilla
1½ cups tightly packed baby arugula
2 tablespoons tarragon leaves
1 avocado, peeled and diced
1 peach, peeled and diced
½ cup thinly sliced Vidalia onion
Kosher or sea salt and freshly ground
black pepper, to taste (optional)

1. In a measuring cup, whisk water, orange juice concentrate, garlic, vinegar, oil, and vanilla together until well mixed.

2. Prepare salad by arranging layers of arugula and tarragon, then avocado, peach, and onions.

3. Drizzle with prepared orange juice vinaigrette. Season with salt and pepper, if desired, and serve.

Experiment Sensibly

When it comes to new herbs and spices, err on the side of caution. Not sure whether or not you like a seasoning? Mix all other ingredients together and test a bite of salad with pinch of herb or spice before adding it to the entire recipe.

Orange-Avocado Slaw

NUTRITIONAL ANALYSIS (per serving, without salt)

Calories: 60   Protein: 2g   Carbohydrates: 5g   Fat: 5g   Saturated Fat: 1g   Cholesterol: 0mg   Sodium: 14mg
Fiber: 2g   PCF Ratio: 11-27-62   Exchange Approx.: 1 Fat, ½ Vegetable

INGREDIENTS | **SERVES 10**

¼ cup orange juice

½ teaspoon curry powder

⅛ teaspoon ground cumin

¼ teaspoon sugar

1 teaspoon white wine vinegar

1 tablespoon olive oil

1 avocado, peeled and chopped

5 cups broccoli slaw mix

Sea salt and freshly ground black pepper, to taste (optional)

1. In a small bowl, whisk together the orange juice, curry powder, cumin, sugar, and vinegar. Add the olive oil in a stream, whisking until emulsified.

2. In a large bowl, toss the avocado with the slaw mix. Drizzle with vinaigrette. Chill until ready to serve. Season with salt and pepper, if desired.

Spinach Salad with Apple-Avocado Dressing

NUTRITIONAL ANALYSIS (per serving)

Calories: 122 Protein: 2g Carbohydrates: 8g Fat: 10g Saturated Fat: 1g Cholesterol: 0mg Sodium: 90mg
Fiber: 3g PCF Ratio: 7-25-68 Exchange Approx.: 2½ Fats, 1 Free Vegetable

INGREDIENTS | SERVES 4

¼ cup unsweetened apple juice

1 teaspoon (or up to 1 tablespoon) cider vinegar

1 clove garlic, minced

1 teaspoon Bragg's Liquid Aminos or soy sauce

½ teaspoon Worcestershire sauce (see recipe for homemade in Chapter 16)

2 teaspoons olive oil

1 avocado, peeled and chopped

2½ cups tightly packed spinach and other salad greens

½ cup thinly sliced red onion

½ cup sliced radishes

½ cup bean sprouts

1. In a blender or food processor, combine the apple juice, vinegar (the amount of which will depend on how you like your dressing), garlic, Liquid Aminos, Worcestershire, oil, and avocado. Process until smooth.

2. In a large bowl, toss the greens, onions, radishes, and bean sprouts.

3. Pour dressing over salad and toss again.

Salads Don't Have to Be Fat-Free

Unless on a calorie-restricted diet, fat-free may not be the best choice—consult your dietitian. Vegetable oils—combined with a diet rich in fish, fruits, vegetables, whole grains, and nuts—are much healthier than using chemically created fat-free foods and are believed to prevent certain cancers, too.

Taco Salad

NUTRITIONAL ANALYSIS (per serving)

Calories: **426**   Protein: **23g**   Carbohydrates: **58g**   Fat: **13g**   Saturated Fat: **7g**   Cholesterol: **30mg**   Sodium: **380mg**
Fiber: **13g**   PCF Ratio: **21-53-26**   Exchange Approx.: **1 Lean Meat, 1 High-Fat Meat, 3 Starches, 2 Vegetables**

INGREDIENTS | SERVES 8

1 recipe Turkey Chili (see Chapter 10)

8 cups tightly packed salad greens

8 ounces Cheddar cheese, shredded (to yield 2 cups)

8 ounces nonfat corn chips

Nonstarchy free-exchange vegetables of your choice, such as chopped celery, onion, or banana or jalapeño peppers (optional)

1. Prepare Turkey Chili.

2. Divide salad greens between 8 large bowls. Top with chili, Cheddar cheese, corn chips, and vegetables or peppers, if using.

Rainbow Potato Salad

NUTRITIONAL ANALYSIS (per serving)

Calories: 146   Protein: 5g   Carbohydrates: 29g   Fat: 2g   Saturated Fat: 0g   Cholesterol: 0mg   Sodium: 615mg
Fiber: 5g   PCF Ratio: 12-77-11   Exchange Approx.: 1½ Starches

INGREDIENTS | SERVES 6

2 pounds red potatoes (6 medium)
⅓ cup finely chopped carrots
¼ cup finely chopped onion
¼ cup finely chopped green pepper
¼ cup finely chopped yellow or red bell pepper
2 tablespoons red wine vinegar
2 tablespoons lemon juice
¼ teaspoon celery seed
1 teaspoon sugar
½ teaspoon salt
2 tablespoons light mayonnaise

1. Wash and scrub the red potatoes. Place whole potatoes in a pot and cover with water. Boil over medium heat for about 20 minutes until potatoes are cooked. Drain and set aside to cool.

2. In a small bowl, combine the carrots, onion, peppers, vinegar, lemon juice, celery seed, sugar, and salt, and mix well. Cover and refrigerate for 2–3 hours.

3. After vegetables have marinated, add light mayonnaise and mix well.

4. Cut potatoes (with skins on) into ½" cubes.

5. In large bowl, combine the potatoes and vegetables and mix well. Chill before serving.

Potato and Snow Pea Salad

NUTRITIONAL ANALYSIS (per serving)

Calories: **139**   Protein: **5g**   Carbohydrates: **28g**   Fat: **1g**   Saturated Fat: **0g**   Cholesterol: **3mg**   Sodium: **223mg**
Fiber: **3g**   PCF Ratio: **13-78-9**   Exchange Approx.: **1 Starch, 1 Vegetable, ½ Fat**

INGREDIENTS | **SERVES 8**

2 pounds red potatoes (6 medium)
3 slices bacon
½ cup chopped onion
¾ pound snow peas, cut in ½" pieces
½ teaspoon salt
¼ cup apple cider vinegar

1. Wash and scrub the red potatoes. Place whole potatoes in pot and cover with water. Boil over medium heat for 20 minutes until potatoes are cooked. Drain and chill. Once chilled, cut into ½" cubes.

2. Cut bacon slices into ½" pieces. Place in nonstick fry pan with the onions and fry for 3–4 minutes until crisp. There should be a light coating of fat in the pan from the bacon.

3. Add the snow peas. Toss with the bacon and onion mixture for 2 minutes. Remove from heat.

4. In a small bowl, dissolve the salt into the cider vinegar. Mix into the snow peas.

5. In large bowl, combine the potatoes and snow peas and mix well.

Summer Salad

Calories: 73   Protein: 2g   Carbohydrates: 7g   Fat: 5g   Saturated Fat: 1g   Cholesterol: 0mg   Sodium: 109mg
Fiber: 2g   PCF Ratio: 9-36-55   Exchange Approx.: 1½ Vegetables, 1 Fat

INGREDIENTS | SERVES 6

2 cups snap peas, cut into 1" pieces

2 cups summer squash, cut into ½" pieces

½ cup chopped carrots

3 tablespoons minced mushrooms

2 cups chopped cucumbers

¼ cup thinly sliced onion

2 tablespoons canola oil

2 tablespoons balsamic vinegar

¼ teaspoon salt

¼ teaspoon thyme

¼ teaspoon marjoram

1. Combine the snap peas, squash, carrots, and mushrooms in medium saucepan with a steamer basket and steam for 2–3 minutes, until crisp-tender. Cool and refrigerate.

2. Once cooled, add the cucumbers and onions.

3. In a small bowl, whisk together the canola oil, balsamic vinegar, salt, thyme, and marjoram. Pour over the vegetables. Toss lightly and serve immediately.

Tip

Add the oil and vinegar dressing just before serving. Minimize the exposure of vinegar to certain vegetables such as snap peas or green beans to retain their bright colors.

CHAPTER 16

Salad Dressings, Salsas, and Sauces

Creamy Feta Vinaigrette

NUTRITIONAL ANALYSIS (per serving)

Calories: **31** Protein: **1g** Carbohydrates: **1g** Fat: **2g** Saturated Fat: **1g** Cholesterol: **4mg** Sodium: **57mg**
Fiber: **0g** PCF Ratio: **17-17-66** Exchange Approx.: **½ Fat**

INGREDIENTS | **YIELDS ABOUT ⅔ CUP; SERVING SIZE: 1 TABLESPOON**

½ cup plain low-fat yogurt
1 tablespoon lemon juice
1 tablespoon olive oil
1½ ounces feta cheese
2 teaspoons mint
½ packet Splenda (optional)
Fresh-ground pepper, to taste

Process all the ingredients in a food processor or blender. Chill before serving.

Bleu Cheese Dressing

NUTRITIONAL ANALYSIS (per serving)

Calories: **24** Protein: **1g** Carbohydrates: **1g** Fat: **2g** Saturated Fat: **1g** Cholesterol: **3mg** Sodium: **52mg**
Fiber: **0g** PCF Ratio: **21-23-57** Exchange Approx.: **½ Fat**

INGREDIENTS | **YIELDS 6 TABLESPOONS; SERVING SIZE: 1 TABLESPOON**

2 tablespoons plain nonfat yogurt
1 tablespoon cottage cheese
1 tablespoon real mayonnaise
½ teaspoon lemon juice
½ teaspoon honey
1 tablespoon plus 2 teaspoons crumbled bleu cheese

1. Place the yogurt, cottage cheese, mayonnaise, lemon juice, and honey in a blender and process until smooth.

2. Fold in bleu cheese.

Raspberry Tarragon Vinaigrette

NUTRITIONAL ANALYSIS (per serving, without salt)

Calories: **120**   Protein: **0g**   Carbohydrates: **9g**   Fat: **9g**   Saturated Fat: **1g**   Cholesterol: **0mg**   Sodium: **0mg**   Fiber: **0g**   PCF Ratio: **0-33-67**   Exchange Approx.: **2 Fats**

INGREDIENTS	YIELDS ¾ CUP; SERVING SIZE: 1 TABLESPOON

½ cup olive oil

¼ cup raspberry vinegar (see recipe in sidebar)

2 teaspoons lemon juice

½ tablespoon finely chopped tarragon

Salt and pepper, to taste

Combine all the ingredients in a covered jar. Shake thoroughly.

Making Raspberry Vinegar

Combine 2 cups raspberries, lightly mashed; 2 tablespoons honey; and 2 cups red wine vinegar in nonstick saucepan. Simmer uncovered for 10 minutes; cool. Place in 1-quart jar and store at room temperature for 3 weeks. Strain vinegar from berries and pour strained vinegar into an empty wine bottle. Cork or cap.

Dijon Vinaigrette

NUTRITIONAL ANALYSIS (per serving)

Calories: 74   Protein: 0g   Carbohydrates: 1g   Fat: 8g   Saturated Fat: 1g   Cholesterol: 0mg   Sodium: 266mg
Fiber: 0g   PCF Ratio: 1-2-97   Exchange Approx.: 2 Fats

INGREDIENTS	YIELDS ABOUT 5 TABLESPOONS; SERVING SIZE: 1 TABLESPOON

1 tablespoon Dijon mustard

½ teaspoon sea salt

½ teaspoon freshly ground black pepper

1 tablespoon red wine vinegar

3 tablespoons virgin olive oil

Put all the ingredients in a small bowl. Mix well using a wire whisk or fork.

The Vinegar-Oil Balancing Act

The easiest way to tame too much vinegar is to add some vegetable oil. Because oil adds fat, the better alternative is to start with less vinegar and add it gradually until you arrive at a flavor you prefer.

Tangy Lemon-Garlic Tomato Dressing

NUTRITIONAL ANALYSIS (per serving)

Calories: 7 Protein: 0g Carbohydrates: 1g Fat: 1g Saturated Fat: 0g Cholesterol: 0mg Sodium: 1mg
Fiber: 1g PCF Ratio: 14-44-42 Exchange Approx.: ½ Free

INGREDIENTS	YIELDS ABOUT ¾ CUP; SERVING SIZE: 1 TABLESPOON

1 tablespoon ground flax seeds

2 cloves garlic

⅛ cup cider vinegar

⅛ teaspoon freshly ground pepper

1 small tomato, chopped

¼ teaspoon celery seed

1 tablespoon lemon juice

¼ cup water

Place all the ingredients in a blender and blend until smooth.

Friendly Fat and Fiber

In addition to providing fiber, ground flax seeds are rich sources of omega-3 and omega-6 essential fatty acids. The oil is low in saturated fat and therefore a heart-healthy choice. Just remember that flax seed oil must be refrigerated or it will go rancid.

Lemon-Almond Dressing

NUTRITIONAL ANALYSIS (per serving)

Calories: 25 Protein: 1g Carbohydrates: 2g Fat: 2g Saturated Fat: 0g Cholesterol: 0mg Sodium: 0mg
Fiber: 1g PCF Ratio: 12-27-61 Exchange Approx.: ½ Fat

INGREDIENTS | **YIELDS ABOUT ⅔ CUP;
SERVING SIZE:
1 TABLESPOON**

¼ cup raw almonds

1 tablespoon lemon juice

¼ cup water

1½ teaspoons honey

¼ teaspoon lemon pepper

½ slice (1" thickness) peeled ginger

¼ clove garlic

1½ teaspoons chopped fresh chives, or
½ teaspoon dried chives

1½ teaspoons chopped fresh sweet
basil, or ½ teaspoon dried basil

Put all the ingredients in a food processor or blender and process until smooth.

Salad: Undressed

Make a quick salad without dressing by mixing chopped celery, onion, and other vegetables such as cucumbers or zucchini. Add low-salt seasoning or toss vegetables with Bragg's Liquid Aminos or low-sodium soy sauce and serve over salad greens.

Caribbean Kiwi Salsa

NUTRITIONAL ANALYSIS (per serving)

Calories: 79   Protein: 2g   Carbohydrates: 19g   Fat: 0g   Saturated Fat: 0g   Cholesterol: 0mg   Sodium: 28mg
Fiber: 3g   PCF Ratio: 9-87-5   Exchange Approx.: 1 Fruit, ½ Vegetable

INGREDIENTS | SERVES 6

1 cup peeled and chopped kiwi
1 cup chopped pineapple
1 cup peeled and chopped mango
⅓ cup chopped red onion
1 cup chopped red bell pepper
⅓ cup black beans, cooked
3 tablespoons chopped fresh cilantro
2 tablespoons lime juice
½ teaspoon chili powder
Dash cayenne

1. Mix all the ingredients together in a medium bowl.

2. Chill for at least 2 hours before serving.

Fresh Peach-Mango Salsa

NUTRITIONAL ANALYSIS (per serving)

Calories: **45** Protein: **1g** Carbohydrates: **10g** Fat: **1g** Saturated Fat: **0g** Cholesterol: **0mg** Sodium: **104mg**
Fiber: **2g** PCF Ratio: **9-82-9** Exchange Approx.: **½ Fruit**

INGREDIENTS | SERVES 6

1 cup mango, peeled and cut into ¼"
pieces

1 peach, peeled and cut into ¼" pieces

1 cup finely chopped red onion

1 cup cucumber, peeled and cut into ¼"
pieces

1 tablespoon balsamic vinegar

1 tablespoon lime juice

1 teaspoon chili powder

½ teaspoon cumin

1 tablespoon chopped fresh cilantro

1 tablespoon chopped parsley

¼ teaspoon salt

1. Mix all the ingredients together in a medium bowl.

2. Chill for at least 4 hours before serving.

Roasted Corn Salsa

NUTRITIONAL ANALYSIS (per serving)

Calories: 104   Protein: 4g   Carbohydrates: 24g   Fat: 1g   Saturated Fat: 0g   Cholesterol: 0mg   Sodium: 77mg
Fiber: 3g   PCF Ratio: 12-80-8   Exchange Approx.: 1 Starch, ½ Vegetable

INGREDIENTS | SERVES 6

2 ears corn

1½ cups fresh tomatoes, skinned and chopped

½ cup chopped red onion

3 tablespoons finely chopped jalapeño pepper

1 tablespoon rice wine vinegar

¼ cup chopped roasted red pepper

1½ tablespoons chopped cilantro

1 teaspoon finely chopped garlic

1 tablespoon lime juice

½ teaspoon cumin

2 teaspoons red wine vinegar

1. Husk the corn and place on a grill. Cook for about 10–12 minutes until lightly browned and tender. Set aside to cool.

2. In a medium bowl, combine the tomatoes, onion, jalapeño, rice wine vinegar, red pepper, cilantro, garlic, lime juice, cumin, and vinegar.

3. When the corn has cooled, cut kernels off cob and add to remaining ingredients. Mix well.

Cranberry Orange Relish

NUTRITIONAL ANALYSIS (per serving)

Calories: 62   Protein: 0g   Carbohydrates: 16g   Fat: 0g   Saturated Fat: 0g   Cholesterol: 0mg   Sodium: 3mg
Fiber: 2g   PCF Ratio: 3-96-1   Exchange Approx.: 1 Fruit

INGREDIENTS | **SERVES 12; SERVING SIZE ½ CUP**

16 ounces fresh cranberries
1½ cups orange sections
2 teaspoons orange zest
¼ cup brown sugar
⅓ cup Splenda Granular
1 teaspoon cinnamon

1. Place the cranberries and orange sections in a food processor and chop using the pulse setting until coarsely chopped. Transfer to a saucepan.

2. Bring cranberry mixture, orange zest, brown sugar, and Splenda to a boil over medium heat. Cook for 2 minutes.

3. Remove from heat, and stir in cinnamon. Chill before serving.

Horseradish Mustard

NUTRITIONAL ANALYSIS (per serving)

Calories: 10   Protein: 0g   Carbohydrates: 1g   Fat: 1g   Saturated Fat: 0g   Cholesterol: 0mg   Sodium: 68mg
Fiber: 0g   PCF Ratio: 12-25-63   Exchange Approx.: 1 Free Condiment

INGREDIENTS | **YIELDS ¾ CUP; SERVING SIZE: 1 TEASPOON**

¼ cup dry mustard
2½ tablespoons prepared horseradish
1 teaspoon sea salt
¼ cup white wine vinegar
1 tablespoon olive oil
Cayenne pepper, to taste (optional)

Combine all the ingredients in a food processor or blender. Process until smooth. Pour into a jar and store in refrigerator. Will last up to 3 weeks refrigerated.

Cranberry-Raisin Chutney

NUTRITIONAL ANALYSIS (per serving, without salt)

Calories: 14 Protein: 0g Carbohydrates: 3g Fat: 0g Saturated Fat: 0g Cholesterol: 0mg Sodium: 1mg
Fiber: 0g PCF Ratio: 4-93-3 Exchange Approx.: 1 Free Condiment

INGREDIENTS | YIELDS ABOUT 3 CUPS;
SERVING SIZE:
1 TABLESPOON

1 cup diced onions
1 cup diced, peeled apples
1 cup diced bananas
1 cup diced peaches
¼ cup raisins
¼ cup dry white wine
¼ cup dried cranberries
¼ cup apple cider vinegar
1 teaspoon brown sugar
Sea salt and freshly ground black
pepper, to taste (optional)

Tip

This chutney is also good if you substitute
other dried fruit for the raisins or cranberries, such as using the dried Fancy Fruit Mix
from Nutty Guys (www.nuttyguys.com).

1. In a large saucepan, combine all the ingredients. Cook
   over low heat for about 1 hour, stirring occasionally.
   Cool completely.

2. Can be kept for a week in refrigerator or in freezer for 3
   months, or canned using same sterilizing method
   you'd use to can mincemeat.

Roasted Red Pepper and Plum Sauce

NUTRITIONAL ANALYSIS (per serving)

Calories: 38   Protein: 0g   Carbohydrates: 10g   Fat: 1g   Saturated Fat: 0g   Cholesterol: 0mg   Sodium: 76mg
Fiber: 1g   PCF Ratio: 3-95-2   Exchange Approx.: ½ Misc. Carbohydrate

INGREDIENTS	YIELDS 2 CUPS; SERVING SIZE: 1 TABLESPOON

1 large roasted red pepper, pulp only (see sidebar)

½ pound apricots, quartered and pitted

¾ pound plums, quartered and pitted

1⅓ cups apple cider vinegar

⅔ cup water

⅓ cup white sugar

½ cup brown sugar

2 tablespoons corn syrup

2 tablespoons fresh grated ginger

1 teaspoon salt

1 tablespoon toasted mustard seeds

4 scallions, chopped (white part only)

1 teaspoon minced garlic

½ teaspoon ground cinnamon

1. Place all the ingredients together in large pot and bring to a boil. Reduce heat and simmer, covered, for 30 minutes.

2. Uncover and simmer for 1 hour.

3. Place in a blender or food processor and process to desired consistency. Can be stored in refrigerator for 4–6 weeks.

Roasting Red Peppers

The traditional method of roasting a red pepper is to use a long-handled fork to hold the pepper over the open flame of a gas burner until it is charred. Of course, there are a variety of other methods as well. You can place the pepper on a rack set over an electric burner and turn it occasionally, until the skin is blackened. This should take about 4–6 minutes. You can also put the pepper over direct heat on a preheated grill. Use tongs to turn the pepper occasionally. Another method is to broil the pepper on a broiler rack about 2 inches from the heat, turning the pepper every 5 minutes. Total broiling time will be about 15–20 minutes, or until the skins are blistered and charred. The key to peeling the peppers is letting them sit in their steam in a closed container until they are cool. Once the peppers are cool, the skin will rub or peel off easily.

Homemade Worcestershire Sauce

NUTRITIONAL ANALYSIS (per serving)

Calories: 14 Protein: 0g Carbohydrates: 4g Fat: 0g Saturated Fat: 0g Cholesterol: 0mg Sodium: 15mg
Fiber: 0g PCF Ratio: 3-97-0 Exchange Approx.: 1 Free Condiment

INGREDIENTS | **YIELDS 1 CUP;**
SERVING SIZE:
1 TABLESPOON

1½ cups cider vinegar

¼ cup plum jam

1 tablespoon blackstrap molasses

1 clove garlic, crushed

⅛ teaspoon chili powder

⅛ teaspoon ground cloves

Pinch of cayenne pepper

¼ cup chopped onion

½ teaspoon ground allspice

⅛ teaspoon dry mustard

1 teaspoon Bragg's Liquid Aminos

1. Combine all the ingredients in a large saucepan. Stir until the mixture boils. Lower heat and simmer uncovered for 1 hour, stirring occasionally.

2. Store in covered jar in refrigerator. Will last in refrigerator up to 3 weeks.

Basil Pesto

NUTRITIONAL ANALYSIS (per serving)

Calories: 37   Protein: 1g   Carbohydrates: 1g   Fat: 4g   Saturated Fat: 1g   Cholesterol: 1mg   Sodium: 14mg
Fiber: 0g   PCF Ratio: 10-6-85   Exchange Approx.: 1 Fat

INGREDIENTS | **YIELDS ABOUT 3 CUPS; SERVING SIZE: 1 TABLESPOON**

¾ cup pine nuts
4 cups tightly packed fresh basil leaves
½ cup freshly grated Parmesan cheese
3 large garlic cloves, minced
¼ teaspoon salt
1 teaspoon freshly ground black pepper
½ cup extra-virgin olive oil

Pesto: Not Just for Pasta!

Although most people use pesto in pasta dishes, you don't have to stop there! Pesto is a versatile sauce that can be added to potatoes, rice, or just about any other grain side dish. For quick and easy seasoning, add it to your next pot of tomato sauce or soup!

1. Preheat the oven to 350°F.

2. Spread the pine nuts on a baking sheet. Bake for about 5 minutes and then stir. Continue to bake for 10 minutes until nuts are golden brown and highly aromatic, stirring occasionally. Let nuts cool completely and then chop finely.

3. In a blender or food processor, combine the basil, pine nuts, cheese, garlic, salt, pepper, and all but 1 tablespoon olive oil. Process until smooth and uniform.

4. Pour into an airtight container and add remaining olive oil on top to act as protective barrier. Pesto can be stored in refrigerator for up to 5 days.

5. To freeze pesto, place it in a tightly sealed container. To freeze small amounts of pesto, pour into ice cube trays and freeze until solid. Once frozen, you can remove the pesto cubes and place them in sealed freezer bags.

Mock Cream

NUTRITIONAL ANALYSIS (per recipe)

Calories: 147   Protein: 14g   Carbohydrates: 21g   Fat: 1g   Saturated Fat: 1g   Cholesterol: 8mg   Sodium: 221mg
Fiber: 0g   PCF Ratio: 39-57-3   Exchange Approx.: 1½ Skim Milks

INGREDIENTS | **YIELDS 1¼ CUPS; SERVING SIZE: 2 TABLESPOONS**

1 cup skim milk
¼ cup nonfat dry milk

Process all the ingredients in a blender until mixed. Use as a substitute for heavy cream.

Comparative Analysis

Using 1¼ cups heavy cream would give you the following breakdown: Calories: 515.02; Protein: 3.06g; Carbohydrates: 4.17g; Fat: 55.27g; Saturated Fat: 34.40g; Cholesterol: 204.79mg; Sodium: 56.16mg; Fiber: 0.00g; PCF Ratio: 2-3-95; Exchange Approx.: 11 Fats.

Fat-Free Roux

NUTRITIONAL ANALYSIS (per serving, roux only)

Calories: 13   Protein: 0g   Carbohydrates: 2g   Fat: 0g   Saturated Fat: 0g   Cholesterol: 0mg   Sodium: 1mg
Fiber: 0g   PCF Ratio: 1-99-0   Exchange Approx.: 1 Free

INGREDIENTS | **YIELDS ENOUGH TO THICKEN 1 CUP OF LIQUID; SERVING SIZE: ¼ CUP**

1 tablespoon cornstarch
2 tablespoons wine

Tip

Make this roux with red wine for a defatted beef broth gravy. Use white wine for chicken or seafood gravy or sauce.

1. Whisk all the ingredients together until well blended, making sure there are no lumps.

2. To use as thickener for 1 cup of broth, heat the broth until it reaches a boil. Slowly whisk cornstarch-wine mixture into broth and return to a boil. Reduce heat and simmer, stirring constantly, until mixture thickens enough to coat back of spoon. (A gravy or sauce made in this manner will thicken more as it cools. It's important to bring a cornstarch slurry to a boil; this helps it thicken and removes the starchy taste.)

Mock White Sauce

NUTRITIONAL ANALYSIS (per recipe)

Calories: 61   Protein: 2g   Carbohydrates: 6g   Fat: 3g   Saturated Fat: 2g   Cholesterol: 9mg   Sodium: 190mg
Fiber: 0g   PCF Ratio: 20-36-44   Exchange Approx.: ½ Fat, ½ Skim Milk

INGREDIENTS | **YIELDS ABOUT 1 CUP; SERVING SIZE: ½ CUP**

1 tablespoon unsalted butter
1 tablespoon flour
¼ teaspoon sea salt
Pinch of white pepper
1 cup Mock Cream (see recipe in this chapter)

1. In a medium-sized heavy nonstick saucepan, melt the butter over very low heat. Butter should gently melt; you do not want it to bubble and turn brown.

2. While the butter is melting, mix together the flour, salt, and white pepper in a small bowl.

3. Once the butter is melted, add the flour mixture, stirring constantly. (A heat-safe flat-bottomed spoon safe for nonstick pans works well for this.)

4. Once mixture thickens and starts to bubble, about 2 minutes, slowly pour in one-third of the mock cream; stir until blended with roux. Add another one-third mock cream; stir until blended. Add remaining mock cream and continue cooking, stirring constantly to make sure sauce doesn't stick to bottom of pan. Once sauce begins to steam and appears it's just about to boil, reduce heat and simmer until sauce thickens, or about 3 minutes.

CHAPTER 17

Salt-Free Spice Mixes

Herbal and Other Seasoning Blends

Using herbs is a delicious way to season dishes and cut the amount of salt needed for flavor, too. Although fresh herbs need to be used immediately, dried herb mixtures can be prepared in advance and stored in an airtight container.

The easiest way to dry fresh herbs is to put them on a baking sheet in an oven at 200–225°F for 1 hour. Blends made from whole seeds or leaves usually need to be coarsely ground in a spice grinder or small food processor prior to using.

Try mixing up a few different spice blends to have on hand. Making your own blends saves time and money. Herbs and spices have no significant caloric value, and since they are made without salt, there is no sodium.

Barbecue Blend

4 tablespoons dried basil
4 tablespoons dried rubbed sage
4 tablespoons dried thyme
4 teaspoons cracked black pepper
4 teaspoons dried savory
1 teaspoon dried lemon peel

Cajun Blend

2 tablespoons paprika
1½ tablespoons garlic powder
1 tablespoon onion powder
½ tablespoon black pepper
2 teaspoons cayenne pepper
2 teaspoons dried oregano
2 teaspoons dried thyme

Caribbean Blend

1 tablespoon curry powder
1 tablespoon ground cumin
1 tablespoon ground allspice
1 tablespoon ground ginger
1 teaspoon ground cayenne pepper

Country Blend

5 teaspoons dried thyme
4 teaspoons dried basil
4 teaspoons dried chervil
4 teaspoons dried tarragon

Fish and Seafood Blend

5 teaspoons dried basil
5 teaspoons crushed fennel seed
4 teaspoons dried parsley
1 teaspoon dried lemon peel

French Blend

1 tablespoon crushed dried tarragon
1 tablespoon crushed dried chervil
1 tablespoon onion powder

Herbes de Provence Blend

4 teaspoons dried oregano
2 teaspoons dried basil
2 teaspoons dried sweet marjoram
2 teaspoons dried thyme

1 teaspoon dried mint
1 teaspoon dried rosemary
1 teaspoon dried sage leaves
1 teaspoon fennel seed
1 teaspoon dried lavender (optional)

Italian Blend

1 tablespoon crushed dried basil
1 tablespoon crushed dried thyme
1 tablespoon crushed dried oregano
2 tablespoons garlic powder

Mediterranean Blend

1 tablespoon dried sundried tomatoes
1 tablespoon dried basil
1 teaspoon dried oregano
1 teaspoon dried thyme
1 tablespoon garlic powder

Middle Eastern Blend

1 tablespoon ground coriander
1 tablespoon ground cumin
1 tablespoon turmeric
1 teaspoon ground cinnamon
1 teaspoon crushed dried mint

Old Bay Seasoning

1 tablespoon celery seed
1 tablespoon whole black peppercorns
6 bay leaves
½ teaspoon whole cardamom
½ teaspoon mustard seed
4 whole cloves
1 teaspoon sweet Hungarian paprika
¼ teaspoon mace

Pacific Rim Blend

1 tablespoon Chinese five-spice powder
1 tablespoon paprika
1 tablespoon ground ginger
1 teaspoon black pepper

Sonoran Blend

1 tablespoon ground chili powder
1 tablespoon black pepper
1 tablespoon crushed dried oregano
1 tablespoon crushed dried thyme
1 tablespoon crushed dried coriander
1 tablespoon garlic powder

Stuffing Blend

6 tablespoons dried rubbed sage
3 tablespoons dried sweet marjoram
2 tablespoons dried parsley
4 teaspoons dried celery flakes

Texas Seasoning Blend

3 tablespoons dried cilantro
2 tablespoons dried oregano
4 teaspoons dried thyme
2 tablespoons pure good-quality chili powder
2 tablespoons freshly ground black pepper
2 tablespoons ground cumin
2 small crushed dried chili peppers
1 teaspoon garlic powder

CHAPTER 18

Breads and Muffins

Basic White Bread

NUTRITIONAL ANALYSIS (per slice)

Calories: 77 Protein: 2g Carbohydrates: 15g Fat: 1g Saturated Fat: 0g Cholesterol: 0mg Sodium: 175mg
Fiber: 1g PCF Ratio: 11-79-10 Exchange Approx.: 1 Starch

INGREDIENTS | **YIELDS 2 LARGE LOAVES; 12 SLICES PER LOAF**

5½–6 cups all-purpose flour

1 package (2½ teaspoons) active dry yeast

¼ cup warm water

2 tablespoons sugar

1¾ cups warm potato water or plain water

2 tablespoons shortening

1 tablespoon sea salt

1. Place ⅓ of the flour in a large bowl and set aside.

2. Mix the yeast with ¼ cup warm water in another bowl, stirring well. Add sugar and potato water to yeast.

3. Add the yeast mixture to the flour and stir well. Set aside for 5 minutes to allow yeast to proof.

4. After 5 minutes, stir the mixture. Cut in the shortening using a pastry blender or your hands.

5. Stir in the salt and as much of remaining flour as possible. Dough has enough flour when it's still somewhat sticky to the touch, yet pulls away from side of bowl as it's stirred.

6. Turn dough onto a lightly floured work surface. Knead for 8–10 minutes, until smooth and elastic, adding flour as necessary. Dough will take on an almost glossy appearance once it's been kneaded sufficiently.

7. Transfer the dough to a bowl treated with nonstick spray. Cover with a damp cloth and place in a warm, draft-free area. Allow to rise until double in volume, about 1–1½ hours.

8. Punch dough down and let rise a second time, until almost doubled in bulk, approximately 30 minutes.

9. Treat two 9" × 5" bread pans with nonstick spray. Punch dough down again and then divide into 2 loaves. Shape loaves and place in bread pans. Cover and let rise until almost doubled, approximately 20 minutes.

10. Preheat the oven to 350°F. Bake for 20–30 minutes. Remove from pans and allow to cool on rack.

Fiber-Enriched Cheddar Bread

NUTRITIONAL ANALYSIS (per slice)

Calories: **141**   Protein: **6g**   Carbohydrates: **25g**   Fat: **1g**   Saturated Fat: **0g**   Cholesterol: **2mg**   Sodium: **546mg**
Fiber: **1g**   PCF Ratio: **19-73-8**   Exchange Approx.: **1½ Starches**

INGREDIENTS | **YIELDS 1 LOAF; 12 SLICES**

1½ cups warm water

1 package (2½ teaspoons) active dry yeast

2½ teaspoons salt

½ cup wheat bran

3 cups bread flour

⅔ cups reduced-fat Cheddar cheese, grated

1 tablespoon Parmesan cheese

Cornmeal, for cookie sheet

1. Combine the water, yeast, and salt in a mixer bowl or food processor.

2. Add the remaining ingredients and mix well using dough hook or dough attachment until very soft dough is formed.

3. Transfer dough to large, loosely covered bowl. Allow to rise at room temperature for 2 hours. Dough can be used after rising, but is much easier to handle after it has been refrigerated several hours or overnight.

4. When ready to bake, sprinkle a light dusting of flour on top of the dough. With floured hands, remove the dough from bowl and shape it into a round loaf.

5. Place the dough on a cookie sheet or pizza peel liberally covered with cornmeal. Allow dough to rise at room temperature for 45 minutes.

6. Preheat the oven to 450°F with baking or pizza stone placed in center rack of oven.

7. Before transferring the dough to the hot stone, slash dough across top using floured sharp knife. Slide dough onto hot baking stone. Place shallow pan of hot water on lower rack of oven to create steam underneath the bread.

8. Bake for 40 minutes, or until bread is deeply browned and has a hardened crust. Remove to a cooling rack and allow to cool before slicing.

Golden Raisin Bread

NUTRITIONAL ANALYSIS (per slice)

Calories: **163**   Protein: **6g**   Carbohydrates: **34g**   Fat: **1g**   Saturated Fat: **0g**   Cholesterol: **0mg**   Sodium: **497mg**
Fiber: **3g**   PCF Ratio: **13-82-5**   Exchange Approx.: **1½ Starches; ½ Fruit**

INGREDIENTS | YIELDS 1 LOAF; 12 SLICES

1½ cups warm water

2½ teaspoons active dry yeast

2½ teaspoons salt

⅓ cup wheat germ

1 cup whole-wheat flour

2 cups bread flour

2 tablespoons honey

1 teaspoon cinnamon

½ cup golden raisins

1 tablespoon egg white

½ tablespoon water

Tools of the Trade

Nonstick pans with dark surfaces absorb too much heat, which causes breads to burn. Chicago Metallic makes muffin, mini-muffin, and other bread pans with lighter-colored Silverstone nonstick coating that are much better suited for baking.

1. Combine the water, yeast, and salt in mixer bowl or food processor.

2. Using a dough hook or dough attachment for food processor, add in the remaining ingredients except the egg white and water. Mix well until very soft dough is formed.

3. Transfer dough to loosely covered large bowl. Allow to rise at room temperature for 2 hours. Dough can be used after rising; however, it is much easier to handle after it has been refrigerated several hours or overnight.

4. When ready to bake, lightly grease a 9" × 4" × 3" loaf pan. Scoop dough out of bowl with wet hands (this makes it easier to handle), shape into elongated loaf, and place in loaf pan. Allow dough to rise for 1 hour.

5. Preheat the oven to 375°F.

6. Brush the loaf with an egg wash of 1 tablespoon of egg white and ½ tablespoon water.

7. Bake on middle rack of preheated oven. Place shallow pan of hot water on the lower rack to create steam under bread.

8. Bake for 45–50 minutes, until bread is golden brown. Cool in pan for 10 minutes, then remove to wire rack. Allow bread to cool completely before slicing.

Whole-Wheat Bread

NUTRITIONAL ANALYSIS (per slice)

Calories: **86** Protein: **2g** Carbohydrates: **17g** Fat: **1g** Saturated Fat: **0g** Cholesterol: **0mg** Sodium: **118mg**
Fiber: **1g** PCF Ratio: **10-77-13** Exchange Approx.: **1 Starch**

INGREDIENTS | **YIELDS 2 LOAVES; 12 SLICES PER LOAF**

1 package (2½ teaspoons) active dry yeast

2 cups warm water

3 cups unbleached all-purpose or bread flour

2 tablespoons sugar

½ cup hot water

2 teaspoons salt

½ cup brown sugar

3 tablespoons shortening

3 cups whole-wheat flour

History Lesson

The sponge process of making bread was more popular years ago, when foodstuffs were less processed and the quality of yeast was less reliable. The yeast works in a batter and the dough rises only once. The sponge process produces a loaf that is lighter but coarser grained.

1. Add the yeast to 2 cups warm water. Stir in all-purpose flour and sugar and beat until smooth, either by hand or with mixer. Set in warm place to proof until it becomes foamy and bubbly, up to 1 hour.

2. In a medium bowl, combine ½ cup hot water, salt, brown sugar, and shortening and stir. Allow to cool to lukewarm. (Stirring sugar until it's dissolved should be sufficient to cool water; test to be sure, as adding liquid that's too warm can kill yeast.) Add to the bubbly flour mixture.

3. Stir in the whole-wheat flour and beat until smooth, but do not knead.

4. Divide the dough into 2 lightly greased pans. Cover and set in warm place until doubled in size, approximately 30 minutes.

5. Preheat the oven to 350°F and bake bread for 50 minutes.

Honey Oat Bran Bread (Bread Machine Recipe)

NUTRITIONAL ANALYSIS (per slice)

Calories: 86   Protein: 3g   Carbohydrates: 16g   Fat: 1g   Saturated Fat: 0g   Cholesterol: 8mg   Sodium: 109mg
Fiber: 1g   PCF Ratio: 15-72-13   Exchange Approx.: 1 Starch

INGREDIENTS | YIELDS 1 LARGE LOAF; 12 SLICES

1¼ cups skim milk

2 tablespoons nonfat buttermilk powder

1 tablespoon olive or canola oil

1 medium egg

1 cup oat bran

1 teaspoon sea salt

½ cup whole-wheat flour

2½ cups unbleached all-purpose or bread flour

1 tablespoon honey

1 package (2½ teaspoons) active dry yeast

Use the light-crust setting on your bread machine. Add the ingredients in the order recommended by manufacturer. Be careful yeast doesn't come in contact with salt.

7-Grain Bread (Bread Machine Recipe)

NUTRITIONAL ANALYSIS (per slice)

Calories: 82   Protein: 3g   Carbohydrates: 15g   Fat: 1g   Saturated Fat: 0g   Cholesterol: 8mg   Sodium: 108mg
Fiber: 1g   PCF Ratio: 14-73-12   Exchange Approx.: 1 Starch

INGREDIENTS | YIELDS 1 LARGE LOAF; 12 SLICES

1¼ cups skim milk

2 tablespoons nonfat milk powder

1 tablespoon olive or canola oil

¾ cup dry 7-grain cereal

½ cup oat bran

1 teaspoon sea salt

2¼ cups unbleached all-purpose or bread flour

½ cup whole-wheat flour

1 tablespoon honey

1 package (2½ teaspoons) dry yeast

1. Add the ingredients to a bread machine in order recommended by manufacturer, being careful that yeast doesn't come in contact with salt.

2. Bake on whole-wheat bread setting on your bread machine (these vary according to manufacturer).

Lactose-Free Bread

When cooking for someone who is lactose intolerant, substitute equal amounts of water or soy milk for any milk called for in bread recipes.

Multigrain Cornbread

NUTRITIONAL ANALYSIS (per serving)

Calories: **124**   Protein: **4g**   Carbohydrates: **20g**   Fat: **3g**   Saturated Fat: **1g**   Cholesterol: **16mg**   Sodium: **220mg**
Fiber: **2g**   PCF Ratio: **12-65-23**   Exchange Approx.: **1 Starch, ½ Fat**

INGREDIENTS | SERVES 16

Nonstick cooking spray
1 egg
2 tablespoons egg whites
3 tablespoons butter, melted
1½ cups low-fat buttermilk
1 teaspoon vanilla
1¾ cups cornmeal
¾ cup whole-wheat pastry flour
1 tablespoon ground flax seed
3 tablespoons Splenda Granulated
1 tablespoon sugar
4 teaspoons baking powder
½ teaspoon baking soda
Pinch salt

1. Preheat the oven to 375°F. Spray an 8" × 8" square baking pan with nonstick cooking spray.

2. In a medium bowl, whisk together the egg, egg whites, butter, buttermilk, and vanilla. Set aside.

3. In a larger bowl, combine the cornmeal, flour, flax seed, Splenda, sugar, baking powder, baking soda, and salt and mix well.

4. Make well in center of dry ingredients and pour in the buttermilk mixture. Mix gently with spoon until all dry ingredients are moistened, but do not overmix.

5. Spoon batter into the prepared pan. Bake for 25–30 minutes, or until center springs back when lightly touched. Cool on wire rack before slicing into pieces.

Don't Have Buttermilk?

Soured milk is a good substitution for buttermilk in baking. To replace 1 cup of buttermilk in a recipe, stir 1 tablespoon of white vinegar or fresh lemon juice into 1 cup of milk. Let the milk stand for 5 minutes, or until milk thickens.

Cheddar Cornbread (Bread Machine Recipe)

NUTRITIONAL ANALYSIS (per slice)

Calories: 102   Protein: 3g   Carbohydrates: 16g   Fat: 3g   Saturated Fat: 2g   Cholesterol: 8mg   Sodium: 172mg
Fiber: 1g   PCF Ratio: 13-63-24   Exchange Approx.: 1 Starch, ½ Fat

INGREDIENTS | YIELDS 1 LARGE LOAF; 12 SLICES

1¼ cups water

1 tablespoon honey

3 tablespoons butter

¼ cup nonfat milk powder

1 package (2½ teaspoons) active dry yeast

2½ cups unbleached all-purpose or bread flour

1 cup yellow cornmeal

1½ teaspoons sea salt

⅔ cup grated Cheddar cheese

1. Use light-crust setting on your bread machine. Add all the ingredients except the cheese in the order suggested by bread machine manual.

2. Process on basic bread cycle according to manufacturer's directions.

3. At beeper (or end of first kneading), add cheese.

Cottage Cheese Bread (Bread Machine Recipe)

NUTRITIONAL ANALYSIS (per slice)

Calories: 76   Protein: 3g   Carbohydrates: 13g   Fat: 1g   Saturated Fat: 1g   Cholesterol: 11mg   Sodium: 114mg
Fiber: 1g   PCF Ratio: 16-68-16   Exchange Approx.: 1 Starch

INGREDIENTS	YIELDS 1 LARGE LOAF; 12 SLICES

¼ cup water

1 cup nonfat cottage cheese

2 tablespoons butter

1 egg

1 tablespoon sugar

¼ teaspoon baking soda

1 teaspoon salt

3 cups unbleached all-purpose or bread flour

1 package (2½ teaspoons) active dry yeast

1. Add the ingredients to bread machine in the order recommended by manufacturer, being careful yeast doesn't come in contact with salt.

2. Bake on white bread setting, light crust. Check bread machine at "beep" to make sure dough is pulling away from sides of pan and forming a ball. Add water or flour, if needed. (Note: You do not want dough to be overly dry.)

Why Breads Need Salt

Salt is only used in bread to enhance the flavor. If salt comes directly in contact with yeast before yeast has had a chance to begin to work, it can hinder the action of the yeast. Keep that in mind when adding ingredients to your bread machine.

Hawaiian-Style Bread (Bread Machine Recipe)

NUTRITIONAL ANALYSIS (per slice)

Calories: 89   Protein: 2g   Carbohydrates: 17g   Fat: 1g   Saturated Fat: 1g   Cholesterol: 11mg   Sodium: 103mg
Fiber: 1g   PCF Ratio: 11-75-14   Exchange Approx.: 1 Starch

INGREDIENTS	YIELDS 1 LARGE LOAF; 24 SLICES

1 egg

½ cup pineapple juice, or ⅛ cup frozen pineapple juice concentrate and ⅜ cup water

¾ cup water

2 tablespoons butter

1 teaspoon vanilla

½ teaspoon dried ginger

1 teaspoon salt

1½ cups unbleached bread flour

2⅛ cups unbleached all-purpose flour

¼ cup sugar

2 tablespoons nonfat milk powder

1 package (2½ teaspoons) active dry yeast

1. Unless instructions for bread machine differ, add ingredients in order listed here.

2. Bake on light-crust setting.

Fiber-Enriched Banana Bread

NUTRITIONAL ANALYSIS (per slice)

Calories: 141   Protein: 5g   Carbohydrates: 25g   Fat: 4g   Saturated Fat: 1g   Cholesterol: 18mg   Sodium: 290mg
Fiber: 3g   PCF Ratio: 12-67-21   Exchange Approx.: 1 Starch, ½ Fruit, 1 Fat

INGREDIENTS | **YIELDS 1 LARGE LOAF; 12 SLICES**

Nonstick cooking spray
½ cup buttermilk
¼ cup wheat bran
1 cup mashed ripe banana
1 egg
¼ cup egg whites
2 tablespoons canola oil
1 teaspoon vanilla
2 tablespoons honey
1¼ cups whole-wheat pastry flour
½ cup all-purpose flour
⅓ cup Splenda Granulated
1 teaspoon baking soda
1½ teaspoons baking powder
½ teaspoon salt

1. Preheat the oven to 375°F. Spray a 9" × 4" × 3" loaf pan with nonstick cooking spray.

2. Place the buttermilk and wheat bran in a medium bowl. Allow the wheat bran to soak for 10 minutes.

3. After 10 minutes, stir in the banana, egg, egg whites, oil, vanilla, and honey.

4. In a larger bowl, sift together the flours, Splenda, baking soda, baking powder, and salt.

5. Add the dry ingredients to the banana mixture. Using a large spoon, stir just until dry ingredients are moistened. Do not overmix.

6. Spoon batter into the prepared loaf pan. Bake for 45 minutes, or until top is lightly browned and inserted toothpick comes out clean. Cool in pan for 10 minutes before removing to wire rack.

Whole-Wheat Zucchini Bread

NUTRITIONAL ANALYSIS (per slice)

Calories: **178**   Protein: **4g**   Carbohydrates: **29g**   Fat: **6g**   Saturated Fat: **1g**   Cholesterol: **25mg**   Sodium: **243mg**
Fiber: **3g**   PCF Ratio: **9-63-28**   Exchange Approx.: **1½ Starches, 1 Fat**

INGREDIENTS	YIELDS 4 MINI LOAVES; 5 SLICES EACH

Cooking spray
2 eggs
2 tablespoons egg whites
½ cup honey
2 cups zucchini, shredded
⅔ cup unsweetened applesauce
⅓ cup canola oil
2 teaspoons vanilla
2 cups whole-wheat pastry flour
1 cup all-purpose flour
¼ cup Splenda Granulated
1 teaspoon salt
2 teaspoons baking powder
1 teaspoon baking soda
2 teaspoons cinnamon
½ teaspoons nutmeg
⅓ cup sunflower seeds, toasted

Variations

For variation to this recipe, ⅓ cup dried cranberries, currants, raisins, or chopped nuts can be added in place of the sunflower seeds.

1. Preheat the oven to 350°F. Spray 4 aluminum mini loaf pans with cooking spray.

2. In a large mixing bowl, beat the eggs and egg whites until foamy. Mix in the honey, zucchini, applesauce, canola oil, and vanilla.

3. In a separate mixing bowl, sift together the whole-wheat flour, all-purpose flour, Splenda, salt, baking powder, baking soda, cinnamon, and nutmeg.

4. Gradually add the dry ingredients to the zucchini mixture. Mix until all ingredients are combined, but do not overmix. Stir in sunflower seeds.

5. Divide batter evenly into the prepared mini loaf pans. Bake for 35–40 minutes, or until tops are browned and inserted toothpick comes out clean.

6. Remove pans to wire rack and cool for 10 minutes before removing bread from pans. Cool completely before slicing.

Applesauce Buckwheat Muffins

NUTRITIONAL ANALYSIS (per muffin):

Calories: **182** Protein: **5g** Carbohydrates: **27g** Fat: **7g** Saturated Fat: **1g** Cholesterol: **24mg** Sodium: **302mg**
Fiber: **3g** PCF Ratio: **11-56-34** Exchange Approx.: **1 Starch, ½ Fruit, 1 Fat**

INGREDIENTS | YIELDS 12 MUFFINS

1 cup buttermilk
½ cup applesauce, unsweetened
¼ cup canola oil
1 egg
2 tablespoons egg whites
2 tablespoons maple syrup
1 teaspoon vanilla
1¼ cups whole-wheat pastry flour
¾ cup light buckwheat flour
¼ cup Splenda granular
1½ teaspoons baking powder
1½ teaspoons baking soda
¼ teaspoon salt
2 teaspoons cinnamon
¼ teaspoon allspice

Crisp Topping (optional):

1 tablespoon Splenda Brown Sugar Blend
¼ teaspoon cinnamon
¼ cup oats
2 teaspoons ground flax seed
1 tablespoon whole-wheat pastry flour
1 tablespoon butter, melted

1. Preheat the oven to 375°F. Prepare a muffin pan with nonstick cooking spray.

2. In a medium bowl, whisk together the buttermilk, applesauce, oil, egg, egg whites, maple syrup, and vanilla.

3. In a separate bowl, sift together the whole-wheat flour, buckwheat flour, Splenda, baking powder, baking soda, salt, and spices.

4. Gradually add the dry ingredients to the liquid mixture. Mix just enough to combine ingredients. Do not overmix. Spoon batter evenly into prepared muffin pan.

5. In a small bowl, mix together all the ingredients for the crisp topping. Sprinkle evenly on top of each muffin.

6. Bake for 20–25 minutes, or until center of muffin springs back when lightly touched. Cool in muffin tin for 5 minutes before removing to wire rack.

Pear Walnut Muffins

NUTRITIONAL ANALYSIS (per muffin, includes optional topping)

Calories: 195 Protein: 5g Carbohydrates: 27g Fat: 8g Saturated Fat: 1g Cholesterol: 24mg Sodium: 289mg
Fiber: 3g PCF Ratio: 11-54-35 Exchange Approx.: 1 Starch, ½ Fruit, 1 Fat

INGREDIENTS | 12 MUFFINS

1 cup buttermilk
3 tablespoons canola oil
1 egg
2 tablespoons egg whites
⅔ cup pears, peeled and chopped
2 tablespoons honey
1¼ cups whole-wheat pastry flour
¾ cup all-purpose flour
3 tablespoons Splenda Granulated
1½ teaspoons baking powder
1½ teaspoons baking soda
¼ teaspoon salt
1 teaspoon cinnamon
¼ teaspoon ginger
⅓ cup walnuts, chopped

Crisp Topping (optional):
1 tablespoon Splenda Brown Sugar Blend
Pinch ginger
¼ cup oats
2 teaspoons ground flax seed
1 tablespoon whole-wheat pastry flour
1 tablespoon butter, melted

1. Preheat the oven to 375°F. Prepare a muffin pan with nonstick cooking spray.

2. In a medium bowl, whisk together the buttermilk, oil, egg, egg whites, pears, and honey.

3. In a separate bowl, sift together the whole-wheat flour, all-purpose flour, Splenda, baking powder, baking soda, salt, spices, and walnuts.

4. Gradually add the dry ingredients to the liquid mixture. Stir just enough to combine ingredients. Do not overmix. Spoon batter evenly into prepared muffin pan.

5. In a small bowl, mix together all ingredients for crisp topping. Sprinkle evenly on top of each muffin.

6. Bake for 20–25 minutes, or until the center of muffin springs back when lightly touched. Cool in muffin tin for 5 minutes before removing to wire rack.

Whole-Wheat Pastry Flour

Whole-wheat pastry flour is a finer grind of soft white wheat. When used in quick-bread and muffin recipes, it delivers more nutrition and fiber than white flour and yields a lighter texture than whole-wheat flour.

Angelic Buttermilk Batter Biscuits

NUTRITIONAL ANALYSIS (per biscuit)

Calories: 74   Protein: 2g   Carbohydrates: 12g   Fat: 2g   Saturated Fat: 1g   Cholesterol: 6mg   Sodium: 55mg
Fiber: 1g   PCF Ratio: 11-64-26   Exchange Approx.: 1 Starch

INGREDIENTS | YIELDS 24 BISCUITS

3 tablespoons nonfat buttermilk powder

2 tablespoons granulated sugar

¾ cup warm water

1 tablespoon active dry yeast

2½ cups unbleached all-purpose flour

½ teaspoon sea salt

½ teaspoon baking powder

¼ cup unsalted butter

¼ cup nonfat plain yogurt

Why Breads Need Sugar

Bread recipes need sugar or sweetener, like honey, to "feed" the yeast. This helps the yeast work, which in turn helps the bread rise.

1. Put the buttermilk powder, sugar, and warm water in a food processor and process until mixed.

2. Sprinkle the yeast over the top and pulse once or twice to mix. Allow mixture to sit at room temperature for about 5 minutes, or until yeast begins to bubble.

3. Add all the remaining ingredients to the food processor. Pulse until mixed, being careful not to over process the dough.

4. Preheat the oven to 400°F.

5. Drop 1 heaping teaspoon per biscuit onto baking sheet treated with nonstick spray. Set tray in warm place and allow biscuits to rise for about 15 minutes.

6. Bake biscuits for 12–15 minutes.

Orange Date Bread

NUTRITIONAL ANALYSIS (per slice)

Calories: **79**   Protein: **2g**   Carbohydrates: **16g**   Fat: **1g**   Saturated Fat: **0g**   Cholesterol: **8mg**   Sodium: **130mg**
Fiber: **1g**   PCF Ratio: **9-80-10**   Exchange Approx.: **1 Starch**

INGREDIENTS | **YIELDS 2 LARGE LOAVES; 12 SLICES PER LOAF**

2 tablespoons frozen orange juice concentrate

2 tablespoons orange zest

¾ cup pitted, chopped dates

½ cup brown sugar

¼ cup granulated sugar

1 cup plain nonfat yogurt

1 egg

1¼ cups all-purpose flour

¾ cup whole-wheat flour

1 teaspoon baking soda

1 teaspoon baking powder

½ teaspoon salt

1 tablespoon vegetable oil

1 teaspoon vanilla extract

1. Preheat the oven to 350°F. Spray 4 mini loaf pans with nonfat cooking spray.

2. In a food processor, process the orange juice concentrate, orange zest, dates, sugars, yogurt, and egg until mixed. (This will cut dates into smaller pieces, too.)

3. Add the remaining ingredients and pulse until mixed, scraping down the sides of bowl if necessary.

4. Divide the mixture between the pans. Spread the mixture so each pan has an even layer. Bake for 15–20 minutes, or until a toothpick inserted into center of loaf comes out clean.

5. Cool bread in pans on wire rack for 10 minutes. Remove bread to rack and cool to room temperature.

Are Your Eyes Bigger Than Your Stomach?

Use mini loaf pans. It's much easier to arrive at the number of servings in the form of a full slice when you use smaller loaf pans. There's a psychological advantage to getting a full rather than half slice.

CHAPTER 19

Reduced-Carbohydrate Desserts

Glazed Carrot Cake

NUTRITIONAL ANALYSIS (per serving)

Calories: **149** Protein: **5g** Carbohydrates: **28g** Fat: **2g** Saturated Fat: **1g** Cholesterol: **42mg** Sodium: **220mg**
Fiber: **2g** PCF Ratio: **13-74-13** Exchange Approx.: **1 Starch, ½ Vegetable, 1 Fruit**

INGREDIENTS | SERVES 9

1½ cups unbleached all-purpose flour

1 teaspoon baking powder

1 teaspoon baking soda

1½ teaspoons cinnamon

¼ teaspoon ground cloves

¼ teaspoon ground allspice

⅛ teaspoon ground nutmeg

1 tablespoon sugar

⅛ cup (2 tablespoons) frozen, unsweetened apple juice concentrate

2 eggs

¼ cup water

2 tablespoons ground flax seed

1 teaspoon vanilla

3 tablespoons nonfat plain yogurt

1 cup canned unsweetened crushed pineapple, ¼ cup of liquid retained

1 cup finely shredded carrots

¼ cup seedless raisins

Glaze

⅛ cup (2 tablespoons) frozen, unsweetened apple juice concentrate

1 tablespoon water

1. Preheat the oven to 350°F. Treat an 8" baking pan with nonstick spray.

2. In a large bowl, sift together the dry ingredients (except sugar) and spices.

3. Using a food processor or mixer, blend sugar, apple juice concentrate, and eggs until well mixed.

4. Stir water and flax seed together in a small microwave-safe bowl and microwave on high for 30 seconds, then stir. (Mixture should be consistency of egg whites; if it isn't, microwave at 15-second increments until it is.)

5. Gradually beat flax seed mixture into the egg mixture, along with the vanilla, yogurt, and ¼ cup pineapple liquid.

6. Stir in the dry ingredients.

7. Fold in the pineapple (drained of any remaining juice), carrots, and raisins.

8. Spoon mixture into prepared pan and bake for 20–25 minutes. Allow cake to cool slightly while you prepare glaze.

9. To prepare glaze: Mix the apple juice concentrate and water until concentrate is melted. (You can microwave the mixture for 15–20 seconds, if necessary.) Spread evenly over the cake.

Mock Whipped Cream

NUTRITIONAL ANALYSIS (per serving)

Calories: 24   Protein: 1g   Carbohydrates: 2g   Fat: 1g   Saturated Fat: 0g   Cholesterol: 1mg   Sodium: 17mg
Fiber: 0g   PCF Ratio: 21-41-38   Exchange Approx.: ½ Fat

INGREDIENTS | YIELDS 3½ CUPS;
SERVING SIZE: 2
TABLESPOONS

1 envelope Knox Unflavored Gelatine
¼ cup cold water
½ cup hot water
2 tablespoons almond oil
3 tablespoons powdered sugar
1 teaspoon vanilla
1 cup ice water
1¼ cups nonfat milk powder

Know Your Ingredients

"Gelatine" is the name of the commercial Knox Unflavored Gelatine product used to make gelatin. Although any unflavored gelatin will work, the nutritional analyses for all recipes are based on the Knox brand.

1. Allow the gelatin to soften in cold water and then pour into blender. Add hot water and blend for 2 minutes, until the gelatin is dissolved.

2. While continuing to blend mixture, gradually add the almond oil, powdered sugar, and vanilla. Chill in freezer for 15 minutes, or until mixture is cool but hasn't begun to set.

3. In a chilled bowl, add the ice water and nonfat milk powder and using a hand mixer or whisk, beat until peaks start to form.

4. Add gelatin mixture to whipped milk and continue to whip for 10 minutes until stiffer peaks begin to form.

5. This whipped topping will keep for several days in refrigerator. Whip again to reintroduce more air into topping before serving.

Chocolate Cheesecake Mousse

NUTRITIONAL ANALYSIS (per serving)

Calories: **83** Protein: **3g** Carbohydrates: **7g** Fat: **5g** Saturated Fat: **2g** Cholesterol: **9mg** Sodium: **47mg**
Fiber: **0g** PCF Ratio: **13-32-55** Exchange Approx.: **½ Skim Milk, 1 Fat**

INGREDIENTS | SERVES 4

1 tablespoon semisweet chocolate chips
¾ cup Mock Whipped Cream (see recipe in this chapter)
1 ounce cream cheese
1½ teaspoons unsweetened cocoa
1 teaspoon vanilla

1. Put the chocolate chips and 1 tablespoon of Mock Whipped Cream in microwave-safe bowl and microwave on high for 15 seconds.

2. Add the cream cheese and microwave on high for another 15 seconds. Whip the mixture until well blended and chocolate chips are melted.

3. Stir in the cocoa and vanilla.

4. Fold in the remaining Mock Whipped Cream. Chill until ready to serve.

Nonfat Whipped Milk Base

NUTRITIONAL ANALYSIS (per serving)

Calories: 290   Carbohydrates: 42g   Protein: 28g   Fat: 1g   Saturated Fat: 0g   Cholesterol: 11mg   Sodium: 310mg
Fiber: 0g   PCF Ratio: 39-59-2   Exchange Approx.: 2 Skim Milks, 1 Carbohydrate

INGREDIENTS	YIELDS ABOUT 3 CUPS

¼ cup nonfat milk powder
⅛ cup powdered sugar
1 cup chilled skim milk, divided
1½ envelopes Knox Unflavored Gelatine

Whipping Methods

Because you don't need to whip the Whipped Milk Base until it reaches stiff peaks, you can use a blender or food processor; however, you won't be whipping as much air into the mixture if you do, so the serving sizes will be a bit smaller.

1. In a chilled bowl, combine the milk powder and sugar and mix until well blended.

2. Pour ¼ cup milk and gelatin into a blender. Let sit for 1–2 minutes for gelatin to soften.

3. In a microwave-safe container, heat the remaining milk until it almost reaches boiling point, about 30–45 seconds, on high.

4. Add the milk to the blender with the gelatin and blend for 2 minutes, or until gelatin is completely dissolved. Chill for 15 minutes, or until mixture is cool but gelatin hasn't yet begun to set.

5. Using hand mixer or whisk, beat until doubled in size. (It won't form stiff peaks like whipped cream; however, you'll notice it will get creamier in color.)

6. Chill until ready to use. If necessary, whip again immediately prior to folding in other ingredients.

Raspberry Yogurt Delight

NUTRITIONAL ANALYSIS (per serving)

Calories: **121**   Protein: **6g**   Carbohydrates: **18g**   Fat: **3g**   Saturated Fat: **2g**   Cholesterol: **12mg**   Sodium: **74mg**
Fiber: **1g**   PCF Ratio: **19-59-22**   Exchange Approx.: **1 Milk, ½ Fat**

INGREDIENTS | SERVES 4; SERVING SIZE ½ CUP

1½ cups plain nonfat yogurt
2 tablespoons Splenda Granulated
4 tablespoons heavy cream
1 tablespoon Splenda Granulated
¼ cup Raspberry Sauce (see recipe in this chapter)

1. Combine yogurt and 2 tablespoons Splenda in a bowl. Chill in the refrigerator.

2. In separate bowl, whip the heavy cream until moderately stiff. Stir in 1 tablespoon Splenda.

3. To make dessert: Gently fold cream into yogurt. Spoon mixture into 4 dessert or parfait cups. Swirl 1 tablespoon prepared Raspberry Sauce into each cup and serve.

Raspberry Sauce

NUTRITIONAL ANALYSIS (per serving)

Calories: 38   Protein: 1g   Carbohydrates: 9g   Fat: 0g   Saturated Fat: 0g   Cholesterol: 0mg   Sodium: 1mg
Fiber: 3g   PCF Ratio: 5-89-6   Exchange Approx.: ½ Fruit

INGREDIENTS | **YIELDS 12 SERVINGS; SERVING SIZE ¼ CUP**

4 cups raspberries
2 tablespoons Splenda Granulated
2 tablespoons honey
1 teaspoon corn starch
½ tablespoon lemon juice

1. Rinse berries and drain. Place berries in a saucepan and mash.

2. Add Splenda and honey and cook over medium heat until mixture reaches a slow boil. Reduce heat and simmer for 10 minutes.

3. Strain berry juice through mesh sieve to remove seeds. Return to saucepan.

4. In a small bowl, mix the cornstarch with the lemon juice until dissolved. Add to the strained berry juice. Bring liquid to a boil, stirring frequently until mixture thickens slightly, about 10 minutes.

5. Cool and store in refrigerator. Use as dessert topping or mixed in yogurt or pudding.

Peach Bread Pudding

NUTRITIONAL ANALYSIS (per serving)

Calories: **164**   Protein: **7g**   Carbohydrates: **23g**   Fat: **5g**   Saturated Fat: **3g**   Cholesterol: **63mg**   Sodium: **175mg**
Fiber: **2g**   PCF Ratio: **16-55-29**   Exchange Approx.: **1 Starch, ½ Fruit, 1 Fat**

INGREDIENTS	SERVES 9; SERVING SIZE: ½ CUP

Nonstick cooking spray
2 cups 1% milk
2 tablespoons butter
2 eggs
⅓ cup egg whites
1 teaspoon vanilla
2 teaspoons cinnamon
⅓ cup Splenda Brown Sugar Blend
6 slices whole-wheat bread, cubed
2 cups peaches, sliced

1. Preheat the oven to 350°F. Spray a 9" × 9" baking dish with nonstick cooking spray.

2. Heat the milk in small saucepan. Add the butter and melt it in the milk. Allow to cool.

3. In a medium bowl, beat the eggs, egg whites, vanilla, cinnamon, and Splenda.

4. Combine the milk and egg mixtures.

5. Place the cubed bread in prepared baking dish. Place sliced peaches on top of bread cubes. Pour egg mixture over bread and peaches.

6. Bake for 40–45 minutes.

Key Lime Pie

NUTRITIONAL ANALYSIS (per serving)

Calories: **203**   Protein: **4g**   Carbohydrates: **29g**   Fat: **8g**   Saturated Fat: **4g**   Cholesterol: **20mg**   Sodium: **331mg**
Fiber: **1g**   PCF Ratio: **8-57-35**   Exchange Approx.: **1½ Starches, 1½ Fats**

INGREDIENTS | SERVES 10; SERVING SIZE: 1 SLICE

1 cup graham cracker crumbs

1 tablespoon Splenda Granulated

2 tablespoons butter, melted

½ teaspoon lime zest

½ cup Splenda Granulated

6 ounces low-fat (Neufchâtel) cream cheese

1 package instant sugar-free vanilla pudding mix

½ cup 1% milk

1 cup lime juice (5 or 6 limes)

1 tablespoon Knox Unflavored Gelatine

1. Prepare the graham cracker crust: Combine graham crumbs and 1 tablespoon Splenda. Add melted butter and mix well. Press crumbs into 9" pie plate with help of flat surface such as bottom of glass. Bake in a 350°F oven for 10 minutes. Remove from oven and cool.

2. In mixer or food processor, combine the lime zest and ½ cup Splenda. Add the cream cheese and process for 30 seconds. Add the pudding mix and milk and blend well.

3. Pour ¼ cup lime juice into a small measuring cup or bowl and heat in the microwave for 1 minute. Add gelatine to the heated juice and dissolve completely.

4. In a small bowl, mix the dissolved gelatin mixture with the remaining lime juice. Pour lime juice into the food processor slowly. Process until all ingredients are well combined.

5. Pour filling into prepared pie shell and refrigerate for 3–4 hours before serving. If desired, top with Mock Whipped Cream (see recipe in this chapter).

Fall Fruit with Yogurt Sauce

NUTRITIONAL ANALYSIS (per serving)

Calories: **126**   Protein: **3g**   Carbohydrates: **26g**   Fat: **3g**   Saturated Fat: **1g**   Cholesterol: **2mg**   Sodium: **48mg**
Fiber: **3g**   PCF Ratio: **10-72-19**   Exchange Approx.: **1 Fruit, ½ Milk**

INGREDIENTS | **SERVES 8; SERVING SIZE: ½ CUP**

2 cups apples, cubed
1½ cups red seedless grapes, halved
1½ cup pears, cubed
2 teaspoons lemon juice
8 ounces light vanilla yogurt
1 tablespoon honey
¼ cup chopped walnuts

1. Combine the apples, grapes, and pears in a medium bowl. Drizzle 1 teaspoon of lemon juice over the fruit to prevent turning brown.

2. In a small bowl, combine the yogurt, 1 teaspoon lemon juice, and honey.

3. Portion ½ cup fruit per serving. Spoon yogurt dressing over fruit and top with chopped walnuts.

Fruit Compote

NUTRITIONAL ANALYSIS (per serving)

Calories: **117**   Protein: **1g**   Carbohydrates: **24g**   Fat: **2g**   Saturated Fat: **1g**   Cholesterol: **3mg**   Sodium: **29mg**
Fiber: **3g**   PCF Ratio: **3-80-17**   Exchange Approx.: **1½ Fruits, ½ Fat**

INGREDIENTS | **SERVES 4; SERVING SIZE: ½ CUP**

2 cups chopped apples

2 tablespoons dried cranberries

6 dried apricots, diced

¼ teaspoon cinnamon

2 tablespoons water

1 tablespoon brandy (optional; if not used, add additional 3 tablespoons water)

1 tablespoon finely chopped walnuts

1. In a small saucepan, combine the apples, cranberries, apricots, cinnamon, water, and brandy.

2. Cook over medium heat until apples are softened, about 10 minutes. Remove from heat and cover for 5 minutes. Stir in walnuts before serving.

Strawberry Ricotta Pie

NUTRITIONAL ANALYSIS (per serving)

Calories: 238   Protein: 10g   Carbohydrates: 27g   Fat: 10g   Saturated Fat: 5g   Cholesterol: 86mg   Sodium: 183mg
Fiber: 1g   PCF Ratio: 18-45-37   Exchange Approx.: 1 Starch, 1 Lean Meat, 2 Fats

INGREDIENTS | SERVES 8; SERVING SIZE: 1 SLICE

2 cups part-skim ricotta cheese
1 cup graham cracker crumbs
1 tablespoon Splenda Granulated
2 tablespoons butter, melted
2 eggs, separated
1 teaspoon lemon extract
2 tablespoons honey
¼ cup Splenda Granulated
¼ cup egg whites
¼ teaspoon cream of tartar
2 cups strawberries, sliced
1 tablespoon cornstarch
2 tablespoons Splenda Granulated
1 tablespoon lemon juice
1 teaspoon balsamic vinegar

1. Place ricotta cheese in a fine mesh strainer lined with coffee filter. Allow excess water to drain from cheese for 2–3 hours.

2. Prepare graham cracker crust: Combine graham crumbs and 1 tablespoon Splenda. Add melted butter and mix well. Press crumbs into a 9" pie plate with help of flat surface such as bottom of glass. Bake in a 350°F oven for 10 minutes. Remove from oven and cool.

3. Prepare the pie filling: In a medium bowl, mix ricotta cheese, egg yolks, lemon extract, honey, and ¼ cup Splenda.

4. In a mixer bowl, beat the egg whites (2 separated plus ¼ cup additional egg whites) with cream of tartar until soft peaks begin to form.

5. Gently fold the egg whites into the ricotta mixture. Turn into the pie shell.

6. Bake at 350°F for 45 minutes, or until mixture is set and top is golden brown. Remove to wire rack and cool completely.

7. Prepare the glaze: In medium saucepan, combine the strawberries, cornstarch, and Splenda until dry ingredients have coated strawberries. Add the lemon juice and balsamic vinegar and cook over medium heat, stirring constantly. Cook mixture for 5–7 minutes, or until cornstarch liquid is clear and gently bubbling. Cool.

8. Spread cooled strawberry glaze on top of cooled pie. Chill until ready to serve.

Summer Fruit Cobbler

NUTRITIONAL ANALYSIS (per serving)

Calories: 152   Protein: 3g   Carbohydrates: 26g   Fat: 5g   Saturated Fat: 0g   Cholesterol: 0mg   Sodium: 248mg
Fiber: 4g   PCF Ratio: 8-65-27   Exchange Approx.: ½ Starch, ½ Fruit, 1 Fat

INGREDIENTS | **SERVES 8; SERVING SIZE: ½ CUP**

Nonstick cooking spray
1½ cups raspberries
1½ cups peeled and sliced peaches
1 cup sliced strawberries
¼ cup sugar
1 tablespoon Splenda
2 tablespoons whole-wheat pastry flour
1 teaspoon cinnamon
¾ cup whole-wheat pastry flour
1 tablespoon sugar
1½ teaspoons baking powder
½ teaspoon salt
2½ tablespoons canola oil
2 tablespoons milk
2 tablespoons egg whites

1. Preheat the oven to 350°F. Spray a 9" × 9" square baking pan with nonstick cooking spray.

2. Place fruit in bottom of the baking dish.

3. In a small bowl, mix the sugar, Splenda, 2 tablespoons flour, and cinnamon. Sprinkle evenly over the fruit.

4. In a separate small bowl, sift together ¾ cup flour, 1 tablespoon sugar, baking powder, and salt. Add the oil, milk, and egg whites and stir quickly until just mixed.

5. Drop dough by spoonfuls over the fruit. If desired, loosely spread dough over fruit. Bake for 25–30 minutes, until dough is golden brown.

Fun Fruits

Any combination of fresh fruit will work well with this recipe. You will need a total of 4 cups of fruit. Fruit suggestions include blueberries, blackberries, peaches, mangoes, or plums. Keep in mind that nutritional analysis will vary somewhat with different fruit combinations.

Baked Pear Crisp

NUTRITIONAL ANALYSIS (per serving)

Calories: 200   Protein: 2g   Carbohydrates: 42g   Fat: 4g   Saturated Fat: 2g   Cholesterol: 8mg   Sodium: 53mg
Fiber: 3g   PCF Ratio: 3-82-15   Exchange Approx.: 1 Fruit, 1 Fat, 1 Starch

INGREDIENTS	SERVES 4; SERVING SIZE: ½ CUP

2 pears
2 tablespoons frozen unsweetened pineapple juice concentrate
1 teaspoon vanilla extract
1 teaspoon rum
1 tablespoon butter
⅛ cup Ener-G Brown Rice Flour
⅓ cup firmly packed brown sugar
½ cup oat bran flakes

1. Preheat the oven to 375°F. Treat a 9" × 13" baking dish or large flat casserole dish with nonstick cooking spray.

2. Core and cut up pears; place them in the prepared baking dish. (Except for any bruised spots, it's okay to leave skins on.)

3. In a glass measuring cup, microwave the frozen juice concentrate for 1 minute. Stir in vanilla and rum and pour mixture over pears.

4. Using same measuring cup, microwave butter for 30–40 seconds, until melted. Set aside.

5. Toss rice flour, brown sugar, and oat bran flakes in a bowl, being careful not to crush cereal. Spread mixture uniformly over pears.

6. Dribble melted butter over top. Bake for 35 minutes, or until mixture is bubbling and top is just beginning to brown. Serve hot or cold.

Baked Pumpkin Custard

NUTRITIONAL ANALYSIS (per serving)

Calories: **130** Protein: **7g** Carbohydrates: **23g** Fat: **2g** Saturated Fat: **1g** Cholesterol: **63mg** Sodium: **89mg**
Fiber: **2g** PCF Ratio: **20-68-12** Exchange Approx.: **1 Milk, 1 Vegetable, ½ Fat**

INGREDIENTS	SERVES 6; SERVING SIZE: ½ CUP

2 cups solid pack or mashed cooked pumpkin

¼ cup sugar

⅓ cup Splenda Granulated

2 teaspoons cinnamon

½ teaspoon ginger

⅛ teaspoon cloves

2 eggs, slightly beaten

¼ cup egg whites

12 ounces evaporated skim milk

Pumpkin Pie

If using this recipe for pumpkin pie, pour filling into a prepared pie shell and bake in a 350°F oven for 40–45 minutes, or until filling is set. The nutritional analysis per serving is: Calories: 244; Protein: 8g; Carbohydrates: 33g; Fat: 9g; Saturated Fat: 3g; Cholesterol: 63mg; Sodium: 206mg; PCF Ratio: 13-33-54. Exchange Approx.: 1 Starch, 1 Milk, 1 Vegetable, 3 Fats.

1. Preheat the oven to 350°F.

2. In a large bowl, mix together the pumpkin, sugar, Splenda, cinnamon, ginger, and cloves.

3. Add the eggs, egg whites, and evaporated milk and whisk until well blended.

4. Pour into 6 custard cups or a 1½ quart casserole dish. Set cups or casserole in large baking pan. Put pan on rack in oven and pour hot water into pan to within ½" of the top of custard.

5. Bake in custard cups for 40–45 minutes, or 1½ quart casserole for 60–70 minutes, until a knife inserted in center comes out clean. Remove immediately from hot water. Serve warm or chilled.

Strawberry Rhubarb Cobbler

NUTRITIONAL ANALYSIS (per serving)

Calories: **138** Protein: **3g** Carbohydrates: **27g** Fat: **3g** Saturated Fat: **0g** Cholesterol: **7mg** Sodium: **223mg**
Fiber: **3g** PCF Ratio: **7-76-17** Exchange Approx.: **½ Starch, ½ Fruit, ½ Fat**

INGREDIENTS	SERVES 9; SERVING SIZE: ½ CUP

Nonstick cooking spray
4 cups chopped rhubarb
2 cups thickly sliced strawberries
¼ teaspoon lemon zest
⅓ cup sugar
¼ cup Splenda Granulated
2 tablespoons cornstarch
2 tablespoons water
¾ cup whole-wheat pastry flour
1 tablespoon sugar
¼ teaspoon ginger
1½ teaspoons baking powder
½ teaspoon salt
2½ tablespoons canola oil
2 tablespoons milk
2 tablespoons egg whites

1. Preheat the oven to 375°F. Spray an 8" × 8" baking dish with nonstick cooking spray.

2. In a mixing bowl, combine the rhubarb, strawberries, lemon zest, sugar, and Splenda.

3. Dissolve the cornstarch in water. Pour over fruit and stir to coat. Place in prepared baking dish. Set aside.

4. In a small bowl, sift together the flour, sugar, ginger, baking powder, and salt.

5. Add the oil, milk, and egg whites and stir quickly until just mixed.

6. Drop dough by spoonfuls over the fruit. If desired, loosely spread dough over fruit. Bake for 25–30 minutes, until dough is golden brown.

Cranberry Pecan Biscotti

NUTRITIONAL ANALYSIS (per serving)

Calories: **98**   Protein: **3g**   Carbohydrates: **15g**   Fat: **3g**   Saturated Fat: **1g**   Cholesterol: **20mg**   Sodium: **39mg**
Fiber: **2g**   PCF Ratio: **10-59-3**   Exchange Approx.: **1 Starch, ½ Fat**

INGREDIENTS | **YIELDS 30 BISCOTTI;
SERVING SIZE: 1 BISCOTTI**

4 tablespoons sweet butter, softened
½ cup sugar
½ cup Splenda Granulated
2 eggs
½ cup egg whites
1 teaspoon vanilla extract
1 teaspoon lemon zest
2½ cups all-purpose flour
⅛ teaspoon salt
½ teaspoon baking powder
½ cup pecans, chopped
½ cup dried cranberries

Exchange List

Food exchange lists can be an important part of arriving at individualized meal plans. To see a full list of foods with their exchange value visit *www.mayoclinic.com/ health/diabetes-diet/DA00077.*

1. In a medium bowl, beat the butter, sugar, Splenda, eggs, egg whites, vanilla, and lemon zest until smooth.

2. In separate bowl, sift the flour, salt, and baking powder.

3. Add the dry ingredients to the liquid ingredients and mix well.

4. Add the pecans and cranberries. Chill dough for 1–2 hours, which makes it easier to handle.

5. Preheat the oven to 350°F.

6. Divide dough in half; shape each half into a slightly flattened 3" × 9" loaf. Place loaves on a greased cookie sheet and bake for 25 minutes.

7. Remove from oven. When cooled enough to handle, cut loaves into ½" slices. Lay out slices on cookie sheet and return to oven for 20 minutes until toasted on bottom.

8. Remove from oven. Turn over and bake for 15 minutes until other side is toasted as well. Remove from oven and cool on wire rack.

Your 10-Week Plan to Kick Pre-Diabetes!

The 10-Week Plan to Kick Pre-Diabetes is designed to help you set modest goals and put what you have learned into practice. Each week has a healthy lifestyle theme along with two suggested goals to help you achieve success.

Week 1: Check Your Portions

Portion control is everything, even when you choose healthy foods! If you eat large portions, you will have trouble controlling your calories. One simple approach to controlling portions is to use the plate method. The concept is designed to help you put together healthy meals in correct portions and distribute carbohydrates evenly in meals. Using the plate method at lunch and dinner, fill half of your plate with vegetables, one-quarter of the plate with starches, and one-quarter of the plate with meat or meat substitute. A serving of milk and fruit are also added to the meal.

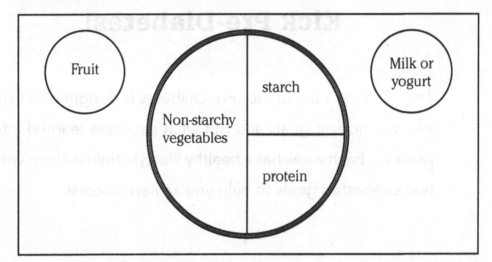

YOUR GOALS FOR WEEK 1
- Give the plate method a try as a means to reduce portion sizes.
- For several days, measure or weigh your food so you can see just how much you are eating.

Week 2: Eat More Vegetables and Fruit Every Day

The recommendation to eat five to nine servings of fruit and vegetables every day sounds like a lot of food, but once you know how to incorporate these foods into your plan it becomes easy. Why that many servings? Because fruit and vegetables are nutrient-dense foods with high fiber and lower calories.

- Take two pieces of fruit from home each day to have for a midmeal snack or with lunch.
- Keep raw vegetables washed, cut up, and ready to eat for quick snacks or salads. If they are there, you will eat them!

Week 3: Get Walking!

Start walking, even if you are only able to manage a few minutes at a time. No matter how long you are able to walk, doing it consistently is most important. Aim for walking most days of the week. Make sure that you have comfortable walking shoes or sneakers.

YOUR GOALS FOR WEEK 3
- Walk for as long as you are comfortably able to. Keep a written record of when and how long you are walking.
- Wear a pedometer so you can track how many steps you take each day. Use the number of steps you take as a motivator to help you increase it each day.

Week 4: Switch to Whole Grains

Begin to switch out the white flour and white grain products in your kitchen for whole-grain foods. Whole grains provide more fiber and nutrients, and have less impact on your blood glucose. Look for products that list whole-grain flour rather than enriched flour as one of the first ingredients.

YOUR GOALS FOR WEEK 4
- Add whole-grain pasta or brown rice to a favorite dish or in combination with vegetables or beans.
- Purchase a new whole-grain food that you haven't used before and try it as a replacement for rice, pasta, or potatoes. Some suggestions: quinoa, kasha, or bulgur.

Week 5: Manage Your Stress

Take stress seriously and find ways to reduce it. Chronic stress can wreak havoc on health and well-being by lowering your immunity and making you more susceptible to many types of illness. You are working on ways to halt pre-diabetes in its tracks; don't let stress derail you!

YOUR GOALS FOR WEEK 5
- Add stretching exercises, meditation, or deep breathing exercises to your daily routine.
- Allow yourself some downtime from the daily grind each day. Make this time for yourself by choosing a relaxing activity that you enjoy.

Week 6: Get Adequate Sleep

Insufficient sleep can have a negative impact on your health. New research has shown that poor quality sleep on a regular basis can contribute to insulin resistance, metabolic syndrome, and diabetes—just what you are trying to avoid!

YOUR GOALS FOR WEEK 6
- Even if you are very busy or have a demanding schedule, resist the urge to skimp on sleep. Make enough time to get seven to eight hours of sleep each night.
- Develop good sleeping habits by rising and retiring about the same time each day. Avoid distractions such as the television at times when you should be going to sleep.

Week 7: Don't Forget the Snacks

Having meals and snacks at regular times can go a long way toward controlling your appetite and blood glucose. Snacking during the day is fine, as long as you make good choices that are low in calories and have nutritional value.

- When you grocery shop, buy healthy snacks to have on hand at all times. Come up with at least two new snack options this week to prevent boredom.
- If necessary, prepare snacks ahead of time, so they are always ready to go, e.g., cut up vegetables, pre-measure nuts into individual containers/baggies, etc.

Week 8: Ramp Up Your Exercise

You may have started an exercise plan several weeks ago, but it's time to take it up a notch. This is important because exercising the same muscles or at the same intensity all of the time will eventually stall your efforts at weight loss.

GOALS FOR WEEK 8
- Turn your moderate walk into a brisk walk. Step up the pace of your walk and add additional steps by using your pedometer to measure your progress.
- Add a few flexibility or weight-bearing exercises to your routine in addition to the walking.

Week 9: Change Your Food Behaviors

Negative food habits are not always easy to change. Make a conscious effort to correct eating habits that cause you to get off track.

GOALS FOR WEEK 9
- Slow down when you eat. Fast eating or mindless eating can cause you to eat too much food before you realize that you've had enough to eat. Place your fork down between each bite and allow more time to eat your meal or snack.
- Drink plenty of water. Take a water bottle with you wherever you go, set one on your desk at work, or find ways to remind yourself to drink more water. Most people need about 64 ounces of fluid a day; make most of it water!

Week 10: Progress Check—Putting It All Together

Monitor your overall progress by looking at how well you have done with various aspects of your plan.

GOALS FOR WEEK 10

- Make a list of all of the things you have been able to achieve, as well as the goals that still need work.
- Seeing in writing all that you have accomplished is very satisfying and motivates you to keep going. Congratulate and reward yourself for a job well done!

Resources

As you learn more about diabetes, you may have more questions or want to find out additional information. The following resources provide a wealth of information regarding diabetes in general, as well as diets, forums, and frequently asked questions.

Online Sources for Diabetes Information

Academy of Nutrition and Dietetics

www.eatright.org

The Academy of Nutrition and Dietetics is the world's largest organization of food and nutrition professionals. This site provides nutrition information and resources on food, food safety, weight management, and a tool to find a dietitian in your area.

American Diabetes Association

www.diabetes.org

This site, maintained by the recognized authority on diabetes, is dedicated to providing up-to-date diabetes information, researching findings, and advocating for people with diabetes.

Ask the Dietitian

www.dietitian.com

Joanne Larsen, MS, RD, LD, maintains this site. You can use it to post specific diet-related questions or read the answers to questions from other visitors.

Changing Life with Diabetes

www.cornerstones4care.com

An interactive website with menu-planning tools, articles, and a free diabetes e-book that you can download.

dLife

www.dLife.com

An interactive diabetes website that includes diabetes information, tips for healthy eating, a recipe bank, and a diabetic community.

National Institute of Diabetes and Digestive and Kidney Disease

www.niddk.nih.gov

Site for general diabetes information, where brochures and articles can be downloaded.

The U.S. National Library of Medicine and National Institute of Health

www.nlm.nih.gov/medlineplus/diabetes.html

This site has research, references, interactive tutorials, consumer materials, and guidebooks to download or order online.

Online Sources for Ingredients and Equipment

The quality of the foods you prepare is based on the quality of the ingredients you use; that's elementary. The equipment you use can make a difference, too. Even if you don't have a gourmet grocery or cooking supply store nearby, you don't have to forego using ingredients or products you've been wanting to try. Chances are you can order them online through one of these sites or find out where products are located near you.

Ancient Harvest

www.quinoa.net

Barilla Plus Pasta

www.barilla.com

Bob's Red Mill

www.bobsredmill.com

Cabot Cheese

www.cabotcheese.coop

Chef's Catalog

www.chefscatalog.com

King Arthur Flours

www.kingarthurflour.com

McCormick Spice

www.mccormick.com

MexGrocer.com

www.mexgrocer.com

Mrs. Dash

www.mrsdash.com

Visit these sites to find a location near you:

Local Harvest

www.localharvest.org

Use this website to find farmers' markets, family farms, and other sources of sustainably grown food in your area, where you can buy produce, grass-fed meats, and many other locally grown foods.

Trader Joe's
www.traderjoes.com

Whole Foods Market
www.wholefoodsmarket.com

For an online food exchange list:

The Mayo Clinic
www.mayoclinic.com/health/diabetes-diet/DA00077

Standard U.S./Metric Measurement Conversions

VOLUME CONVERSIONS	
U.S. Volume Measure	Metric Equivalent
⅛ teaspoon	0.5 milliliters
¼ teaspoon	1 milliliters
½ teaspoon	2 milliliters
1 teaspoon	5 milliliters
½ tablespoon	7 milliliters
1 tablespoon (3 teaspoons)	15 milliliters
2 tablespoons (1 fluid ounce)	30 milliliters
¼ cup (4 tablespoons)	60 milliliters
⅓ cup	90 milliliters
½ cup (4 fluid ounces)	125 milliliters
⅔ cup	160 milliliters
¾ cup (6 fluid ounces)	180 milliliters
1 cup (16 tablespoons)	250 milliliters
1 pint (2 cups)	500 milliliters
1 quart (4 cups)	1 liter (about)

WEIGHT CONVERSIONS	
U.S. Weight Measure	Metric Equivalent
½ ounce	15 grams
1 ounce	30 grams
2 ounces	60 grams
3 ounces	85 grams
¼ pound (4 ounces)	115 grams
½ pound (8 ounces)	225 grams
¾ pound (12 ounces)	340 grams
1 pound (16 ounces)	454 grams

OVEN TEMPERATURE CONVERSIONS	
Degrees Fahrenheit	Degrees Celsius
200 degrees F	95 degrees C
250 degrees F	120 degrees C
275 degrees F	135 degrees C
300 degrees F	150 degrees C
325 degrees F	160 degrees C
350 degrees F	180 degrees C
375 degrees F	190 degrees C
400 degrees F	205 degrees C
425 degrees F	220 degrees C
450 degrees F	230 degrees C

BAKING PAN SIZES	
U.S.	Metric
8 x 1½ inch round baking pan	20 x 4 cm cake tin
9 x 1½ inch round baking pan	23 x 3.5 cm cake tin
11 x 7 x 1½ inch baking pan	28 x 18 x 4 cm baking tin
13 x 9 x 2 inch baking pan	30 x 20 x 5 cm baking tin
2 quart rectangular baking dish	30 x 20 x 3 cm baking tin
15 x 10 x 2 inch baking pan	30 x 25 x 2 cm baking tin (Swiss roll tin)
9 inch pie plate	22 x 4 or 23 x 4 cm pie plate
7 or 8 inch springform pan	18 or 20 cm springform or loose bottom cake tin
9 x 5 x 3 inch loaf pan	23 x 13 x 7 cm or 2 lb narrow loaf or pate tin
1½ quart casserole	1.5 liter casserole
2 quart casserole	2 liter casserole

Index

Note: Page numbers in **bold** indicate recipe category lists.